TREATING THE DISORDER, TREATING THE FAMILY

TREATING THE DISORDER, TREATING THE FAMILY

EDITED BY JIM ORFORD

THE JOHNS HOPKINS UNIVERSITY PRESS
BALTIMORE

© 1987 Jim Orford
All rights reserved
Printed and bound in Great Britain

First published 1987
The Johns Hopkins University Press
701 West 40th Street
Baltimore, Maryland 21211

Library of Congress Cataloging-in-Publication Data

Treating the Disorder, Treating the Family.

Includes index.
1. Mentally ill — Family relationships. 2. Sick —
Family relationships. I. Orford, Jim. [DNLM: 1. Chronic
disease. 2. Family. 3. Mental disorders. 4. Stress,
psychological. WM 172 T784]
RC455.4.F3T73   1987   362.1   87-3159
ISBN 0-8018-3536-4

Contents

Acknowledgements

The editor's grateful thanks go to all who have contributed to this book, and in particular to chapter authors, all of whom responded so positively to my often finicky editorship, and to Liz Mears without whose invaluable assistance at all stages I could not have coped.

Exeter   JIM ORFORD
November 1986

Contributors

Birchwood, Max,
Principal Clinical
Psychologist,
Department of Clinical
Psychology and Family
Centre for Advice, Resources
& Education,
All Saints Hospital,
Winson Green, Birmingham.

Dobash, R. Emerson,
Reader,
Department of Sociology,
University of Stirling,
Stirling.

Dobash, Russell P.,
Lecturer,
Department of Sociology,
University of Stirling,
Stirling.

Eiser, Christine,
Research Fellow,
Department of Psychology,
University of Exeter.

Gilhooly, Mary L.M.,
Lecturer,
Behavioural Sciences Group,
University of Glasgow.

Hay, William,
Director, Behavior Therapy
Center,
The Office Center at
Princeton Meadows,
New Jersey,
USA.

Kuipers, Liz,
Lecturer in Clinical
Psychology,
Institute of Psychiatry and
Honorary Principal Clinical
Psychologist,
Maudsley Hospital,
London.

McCrady, Barbara S.,
Associate Professor of
Psychology and Clinical
Director,
Center of Alcohol Studies,
Rutgers,
The State University of New
Jersey,
USA.

Marshall, Pamela,
Research Nurse,
Leicester General Hospital,
Gwendolen Road,
Leicester.

Moffat, Nick,
Principal Clinical
Psychologist,
District Psychology Service,
East Dorset Health
Authority.

Nichols, Keith A.,
Lecturer,
Department of Psychology,
University of Exeter and
Principal Clinical
Psychologist,
Exeter Renal Unit.

Oppenheimer, Rhoda,
Senior Psychiatric Social
Worker (Teaching),
Leicestershire Social Services
and Leicester University
Department of Psychiatry.

Orford, Jim,
Senior Lecturer in Clinical
Psychology,
University of Exeter,
and Top Grade Psychologist,
Exeter Health Authority.

Pahl, Jan,
Senior Research Fellow,
Health Services Research
Unit,
University of Kent at
Canterbury.

Palmer, Robert L.,
Senior Lecturer in Psychiatry
and Honorary Consultant
Psychiatrist,
University of Leicester and
Leicester General Hospital,
Leicester.

Quine, Lyn,
Research Fellow, Institute of
Social and Applied
Psychology,
University of Kent at
Canterbury.

Smith, Joanne,
Senior Clinical Psychologist,
Department of Clinical
Psychology and Family
Centre for Advice, Resources
& Education,
All Saints Hospital,
Winson Green,
Birmingham,
and Research Associate,
Department of Psychology,
University of Birmingham.

1

Introduction

Jim Orford

A little bit of very personal reminiscence may help to explain my motives for putting this book together and may assist in appreciating its general orientation. Although I was not aware of it at the time, the idea for this book had started to develop in the early 1970s when I was preparing a literature review on the influence of family factors on the outcome of treatment for alcohol problems. With characteristic wisdom my supervisors, Bram Oppenheim and Griffith Edwards, encouraged me to look not only at what had been written about marriage, the family and alcohol problems, but also at the parallel literature on other forms of psychiatric disorder such as depression, and further still to look at the effects upon the family of social crises such as unemployment and separation due to military service.

What I discovered in writing my review was that many of the features of family life that I had assumed to be characteristic of those families with a serious alcohol problem — conflict, poor communication, misunderstanding, a poor sex life, a rearrangement of family roles, heightened anxiety in all family members — were in fact not special to this group of families at all, but were characteristics general to families in distress or disorder for one reason or another. To give just two examples: I was struck by the way in which family members who later came to understand that a member of their family was suffering from 'mental illness' had gone through the same kind of lengthy process of uncertainty about what was wrong (Clausen and Yarrow, 1955) as had been described for families of 'alcoholics'; and I was intrigued by the difficulties that families had in readjusting their roles on the husband's return at the end of World War II (Hill, 1949) which was so reminiscent of descriptions of the difficulties that many families had of readjusting to having a sober husband after many years of excessive drinking. It was as a result of finding a whole series of such parallel observations that I wrote an article entitled 'Alcoholism and marriage: the argument against specialism', which was published in the *Journal of Studies on Alcohol* (1975). The present volume is a direct consequence of that initial shock to my naive assumption that all the difficulties observed in families with alcohol problems were special to them alone.

My principal motive in editing this volume has been to explore the commonalities that exist in the experiences of families that are troubled by a variety of apparently very different disorders, illnesses and handicaps. It seemed to me that others might also be led into making the same mistake that I had made. I began to see other specialisms developing. I wondered if those who were discovering the stresses upon families caring for elderly relatives with dementia, and who were attempting to help them, knew about work on how families attempt to cope with excessive drinking in the family. I suspected that the work of the social psychiatrists on 'expressed emotion' in families, and its influence on relapse in relatives suffering from schizophrenia or depression, was being pursued without due acknowledgement to work in parallel fields. I knew that the impact upon parents of bringing up a handicapped child had been of interest for some while (Tizard and Grad, 1961) but I wondered whether this, like alcohol and the family, was in danger of becoming a speciality. I was aware, also, of growing interest in the impact upon family members of chronic physical illness, either in adults or children, and in the ways families cope with these circumstances. Again I was interested to know how much of the experience of these families was unique and how much was shared with families coping with psychological disorders or handicaps.

At the same time as these specialisms — or fields of knowledge that are in danger of becoming specialisms — have been developing, there has been a general development in the provision of services, away from institutions and towards 'community care'. This has inevitably led to a greater level of concern with the impact of chronic illness, handicap or disorder upon close relatives, with the way they cope, and with their needs. Developing understanding and ways of helping families in these predicaments has long been an essential part of social work, and this now constitutes an important element in a number of emerging sub-disciplines such as community psychology, community psychiatric nursing, community psychiatry and community occupational therapy. There has also been occurring a rapid growth in research on family functioning and in the development of theories of family life (Gale and Vetere, 1987). One way and another professionals and others who have dealings with illness, handicap or disorder are becoming much more alert to the family as part of the social context in which human difficulties occur. There is an eagerness to work with families.

A word is in order about the theoretical orientation of many of the chapters in this book, including the final chapter, which will not please some readers whose orientations towards the family are different. Indeed it was a second driving motive behind compiling this book that it should make a contribution towards correcting some prevailing professional theories about families and disorder which I felt were continuing to stand in the way of helping relatives and involving them fully. More will be said about this in the concluding chapter. Suffice it to say here that it is surprisingly common to find professionals blaming relatives for their families' difficulties, failing to include them, and cutting them off from information. Some early theories of disorder in the family — the 'schizophrenogenic' mother, the dominant wife of an 'alcoholic', or the over-protective parent of a handicapped child, for example — can be seen now to have been crude. Yet they continue to exert a surprisingly strong influence upon professional training and practice. More sophisticated theories which are now in vogue, such as those based upon General System Theory, may be in danger of perpetuating some of the same attitudes by implying that disorder is a symptom of family pathology.

Perspectives adopted by authors of chapters in this book range from the feminist view of Dobash and Dobash in their chapter on marital violence, to the Systems view to which Palmer, Oppenheimer and Marshall give sympathetic attention in their chapter on anorexia. The perspective that readers will meet most frequently in this book, however, is one that Birchwood and Smith refer to in their chapter as a 'transactional' model. According to this perspective it is correct to think of 'disorder' — taken to mean any one of a whole range of family troubles, difficulties, illnesses or handicaps including those considered in this book — as being located in one particular member of the family. When working with this model the identification of one family member as the ill, handicapped or disordered person in the family is accepted by those working with the family, at least as an initial working hypothesis. In this important respect the prevailing view adopted in this book parts company with some Systems perspectives.

The view taken by most authors here is that the family is, nevertheless, to be seen as a complex interacting system. Those attempting to assist from outside meet a family that is very likely to have

3

had a lengthy history, and in many cases a long period of attempting to adjust to disorder. The picture which the family presents is one that has been influenced by the genetic endowments and previous environments of all of its members; by influences from the external environment including accommodation, employment, neighbours, kin who are not living under the same roof, and values and attitudes which prevail in the particular society in which the family lives at that particular historical epoch. Most important of all, the family has been influenced by the continuing process of mutual, reciprocally influential patterns of change and adjustment which are common to all social systems (Bronfenbrenner, 1979).

This transactional process takes on a particularly salient form in the context of families coping with disorder. Family members are not merely victims of the stress caused by living with a relative who is brain-damaged or who drinks excessively, for example. By their attitudes or actions family members inevitably modify the behaviour of the family member identified as possessing the disorder or causing the family difficulty, and the impact of disorder is affected thereby. In some cases relatives may unwittingly help to maintain disorder or some of the problems associated with it.

This is *not* the same as saying that the family has caused a problem. The particular pattern of family interaction which is to be seen by the time outside help is involved is something that has evolved or emerged over time. It is the result of the family's attempts to accommodate to the presence of disorder in its midst. In some instances — in some cases of anorexia or depression for example — the disorder may itself be part of the family's way of accommodating to pre-existing tensions. Even then, however, the picture seen by the professional or outside helper will be largely determined by the efforts of the family to cope with the disorder itself.

There is a multitude of definitions of the word 'system'. The perspective outlined briefly above makes a distinction between just two of them. It views families coping with disorder as a system but not a System: as a group of people whose way of accommodating to disorder in one of its members has emerged over time as a result of a transactional process, but not as individuals with a group pathology or disturbance of which disorder in one member is a symptom.

The content of the book is intended to be representative of the diversity of types of family difficulty for which this perspective is appropriate. Needless to say it is not exhaustive. Three gaps of which

I am very aware are families and drug misuse (Stanton, 1979), families and agoraphobia (Hafner, 1977) and families and unemployment. Readers will doubtless be able to think of other topics which should have been included.

As it is, the book includes chapters on topics which have, between them, been construed as psychiatric or psychological problems, medical illnesses, chronic handicaps or social problems. In terms of age group the disorders considered cover those that affect children, as well as those affecting younger, middle-aged and elderly adults. The temptation to arrange chapters in an apparently logical order was resisted. It was felt that this would be inconsistent with the main intention of the book, which is to explore similarities and differences between families coping with different types of trouble irrespective of factors such as age or conventional categorisation.

Each of the chapter authors is an expert in her or his own field. A number of disciplines are represented, although psychology, and to a lesser extent sociology, predominate. Some authors have developed their expertise as a result of their experience in helping individual families, some by carrying out much-needed research in which families have had an opportunity to speak for themselves, and others have done both. What is common to them all is an unusually detailed and well-informed knowledge about families attempting to cope with a particular problem, and a welcome understanding of the lives and experiences of the families they have tried to help or understand.

REFERENCES

Bronfenbrenner, U. (1979) *The ecology of human development: experiments by nature and design*, Harvard University Press, Cambridge, Massachusetts

Clausen, J.A. and Yarrow, M.R. (1955) The impact of mental illness on the family, *Journal of Social Issues, 11*, 3–65

Gale, A. and Vetere, A. (1987) Some theories of family behaviour. In A. Vetere and A. Gale (eds), *Ecological studies of family life*, Wiley, Chichester and New York (In press)

Hafner, R.J. (1977) The husbands of agoraphobic women and their influence on treatment outcome, *British Journal of Psychiatry, 131*, 289–94

Hill, R. (1949) *Families under stress: adjustment to the crisis of war separation and reunion*, Harper and Row, New York

Orford, J. (1975) Alcoholism and marriage: the argument against specialism, *Journal of Studies on Alcohol, 36*, 1537–63

Stanton, M.D. (1979) Family treatment approaches to drug abuse problems:

a review, *Family Process, 18,* 251–80

Tizard, J. and Grad, J. (1961) *The mentally handicapped and their families,* Oxford University Press, Oxford

2

Schizophrenia and the Family

Max Birchwood and Joanne Smith

The 1960s witnessed a period of great optimism in the treatment of schizophrenia. The introduction of effective forms of drug treatment and prophylaxis led to an increase in the numbers of individuals discharged from hospital and maintained in the community. However in recent years the limitations of this policy have become apparent. The neuroleptic drugs do not always abolish the symptoms; they carry with them a high risk of relapse (50 per cent over 2 years) and social impairment, and frequently lead to distressing side-effects. It was not anticipated at the inception of this policy that many of those discharged into the community would continue to be so impaired and thus, even today, there continues to be a paucity of community resources to meet their needs. The consequence has been that the major burden of care has fallen on the immediate family.

Somewhere in the region of 60–70 per cent of people with schizophrenia will return to live with their families, particularly in the early years following the first admission to hospital (Goldman, 1980). Thus, families occupy a central role in the long-term community care of schizophrenia, a disorder which frequently leads to life-long disability in the young people whom it primarily affects.

Until recently the extent of the burden facing families and the nature of their specific needs have not been recognised by the mental health services. This was due in part to the *Zeitgeist* of the 1960s, which spawned the view that families were instrumental in the genesis of the disorder. For a long time an atmosphere of suspicion and mistrust has reigned between families and the psychiatric services, and consequently families' pleas for help have tended to fall on deaf ears. In this chapter we will argue that a careful consideration of family needs and the options available for helping suggest that a major diversion of money and manpower is necessary in order to train and support families who are maintaining what is often a long-term burden. This offers the prospect not only of alleviating the family burden itself, but also of making a genuine impact on the outlook for this, the most debilitating of the psychiatric disorders.

IMPACT ON FAMILY LIFE

Perhaps the most significant effect on family life comes from the sometimes profound and long-lasting changes in the behaviour of the affected individual.

Table 2.1: Behaviours observed by relatives of acute* schizophrenic individuals living at home

	Percentage observing
Withdrawal	51
Staying in bed	
Emotional detachment	
Avoiding social contact	
Psychotic symptoms	36
Expressing passivity ideas	
Persecutory delusions	
Hallucinatory behaviour	
Behavioural excesses	31
Aggression to relatives	
Restlessness	
Provoking family discord	
Impaired social performance	51
Self-care	
Domestic tasks	
Independence skills	

*Mean age = 26 years; mean admissions = 1.7; mean illness duration = 2.2 years ($N = 53$)

Table 2.1 documents the kind of behavioural changes which were observed by relatives of individuals with acute schizophrenia in a study by the first author. Taking all behaviours into account it was found that some 70 per cent of the families experienced some behavioural disturbance, with particularly severe disturbance in a sub-group of about 15 per cent (similar to the findings of Gibbons, Horn, Powell and Gibbons (1984) and Hewitt (1983)). As far as social performance is concerned Gibbons *et al.* report that at least three-quarters of their sample played only a limited part in household care and management, had limited spare-time activities and gave little support or affection to the main supporter.

The effect on the main supporters, and on family life in general, hinges on the nature and severity of the disturbance in behaviour: the more severe the disturbance, and the more dependent the individual becomes, the greater and more pervasive the impact will tend to be. This impact is usually felt at a number of overlapping levels, which are summarised in Table 2.2.

Table 2.2: Consequences of schizophrenia for family life

Family-patient relationship
    Coping with disturbed behaviour
    Re-establishing the relationship

Emotional changes
    Coping with 'loss'
    Stress symptoms
    Negative emotions: guilt, fear, embarrassment, anger

Family relationships
    Intra-familial tension: arguments, jealousies, divisions
    Loss of cohesion
    Rejection of the individual

Hardship
    Financial/employment problems
    Sacrificing personal needs
    Disruption/dismissal of long-term plans
    Disruption of household routine

It may be readily appreciated that the changes in behaviour and personality can prove extremely distressing for close family members. On the one hand there is the difficult emotional adjustment in coming to terms with the disintegration of the personality in a family member. On the other, the behavioural problems can prove extremely taxing to cope with and, in time, can lead to intra-familial tension, ambivalence in the relationship and sometimes outright rejection. It is clear from studies such as Gibbons *et al.* (1984) that the kind of behaviour which relatives find most distressing and difficult to cope with is that which is directed at them (e.g. rudeness, aggression), or is the product of active psychosis. The following extract from an interview illustrates the difficulty relatives have in knowing how best to respond to this kind of behaviour and the stress and conflict which is aroused in relatives when the disturbance impinges directly on them. The interviewee is the mother of a young person with schizophrenia discussing her reaction to her son's accusations that she is trying to poison him:

the worst of it is the hate in his eyes, sometimes I don't know how he thinks we could do something like that . . . I know he's ill but sometimes I get angry inside, I mean, how would you react if your son said that to you? . . . it's difficult to know what to say to him . . . if you say you're not [poisoning him] that's what he expects. We tried to tell him it was his illness but he just laughed (taken from Birchwood, 1983)

When relatives are asked about their needs, high on their priorities is a concern for advice and guidance about behavioural management (e.g. Kint, 1977). There are often no universal solutions to management questions, only 'best' answers for individual families. It often takes a long period of arduous trial and error before this is appreciated, if ever. One family, for example, went to great lengths to refute their son's ideas that he was 'under observation'. After prolonged argument and debate, his parents realised that refutation of these ideas was impossible: they discovered that it required very little in the way of evidence to support the delusion, as even everyday events were illogically taken as proof (in this case 'enemy agents' occupied red cars and since red cars frequently passed by, this was proof of the conspiracy). As a result this family became somewhat detached from the delusions with clear benefits to their own well-being. Too many relatives fail to achieve this kind of accommodation or 'control' over their situation, or do so only after a long period.

There are numerous emotional responses which can be identified. Guilt is one strong and prevalent emotion which in some instances motivates compensatory over-involvement. The meaning of this guilt is sometimes difficult to discern. Occasionally it seems to be associated with the feeling of uncontrollability; relatives feel they *could* and *should* be doing more, but feel they do not have the resources to manage more effectively. In others the meaning of the guilt stems from the way in which the problem is construed. The psychological character of the disorder raises the concern that early relationships or childrearing practices may be to blame, no doubt influenced by 'pop' psychology.

We have concentrated the discussion so far on the 'key' relative — the parent, spouse or 'significant other' — and referred only obliquely to the family as a set of relationships.

A common cause of intra-familial strife occurs when there is a lack of cohesion between parents or other family members in terms of the way in which the individual and the disturbed behaviour is construed and when family members disagree about how the individual should be managed. This can present a very disturbed and complicated picture. Take for example the following family.

The Dawson family

James has a 3-year history of schizophrenia. He is maintained at home with the support of large doses of neuroleptic medication but he is actively hallucinated and deluded, and believes his sisters are talking about him and plotting against him. James often shouts at the neighbours who he believes to be part of the 'conspiracy'. He is frightened to venture outside the home and spends nearly all of his time in his bedroom where his meals are brought to him. James constantly provokes and accuses his younger sister Marcia, and has hit out at her on more than one occasion. Marcia shouts and swears at James whenever she is approached; however her elder sister Christine manages to stand up to him and therefore it was felt that James exploits the 'weakest link'. Mrs Dawson has been struck on many occasions but tends to remain calm and tells James that she will not sit and talk with him in the evening if he treats her in this way. Unlike his wife, Mr Dawson is ambivalent toward James, who he believes to be malicious; thus Mr Dawson is very punitive toward James. Mr Dawson has a 'soft spot' for Marcia, which she exploits such that she over-reacts to James's behaviour knowing that her father will come immediately to her defence. Conflict has arisen between parents because of Mr Dawson's aggressive style and the father-daughter axis which has developed. These two factors are probably responsible for accentuating James's behaviour and much of the family conflict.

In this family, as in many others, affiliative ties have been weakened and family cohesion impaired.

Descriptive accounts of families' attempts to cope with the emergence of schizophrenia show that many find themselves unable to pursue their interests, social life or other sources of satisfaction as their energies are consumed thinking, worrying and caring for the individual (Creer and Wing, 1973). This sacrifice of personal needs is difficult to avoid and occurs to some degree in most families but in its extreme seems to be positively motivated. In some cases guilt may be aroused ('How can I possibly go out and enjoy an evening with friends when she's sitting at home plagued by voices?'). In others, relatives may feel that the individual is unable to manage alone for short periods and consequently is never given the *opportunity* to do so. This quasi-superstitious situation can tie relatives down unnecessarily. It is not uncommon, for example, to find relatives who have cut themselves off from friends or family, who have few sources of satisfaction and feel unable to take a break.

HOW DO FAMILIES COPE WITH SCHIZOPHRENIA?: FIVE INTERACTING DIMENSIONS OF FAMILY COPING BEHAVIOUR

1. Managing 'schizophrenic' disturbance

The coping strategies adopted by close relatives of individuals with schizophrenia were examined directly in a study of families of young acute schizophrenic patients with a 2-year history of schizophrenia (Birchwood, 1983). These families were experiencing a range of disturbed behaviours and were trying to adjust to their new situation. These families were interviewed at some length about their coping strategies in relation to each kind of behavioural change they witnessed. These individual coping responses fell into a number of groupings or strategies which individual relatives seemed to adopt with some consistency across all behaviours observed:

> *Coercion* is a strategy where the relative adopts a punitive approach including criticism, verbal or physical aggression, threats, attempts to shame or embarrass and idiosyncratic reactions which are intended to provoke confrontation.
> *Avoidance* strategies include responses which minimise relatives' exposure to the behaviour either through withdrawing from the situation or through the adoption of expedients to curtail the behaviour (e.g. relatives might complete tasks with which the individual shows some difficulty).
> *Indifferent* reactions are those where relatives do not respond because they do not perceive the behaviour as a problem; because the behaviour is 'accepted' (e.g. as part of the personality or illness) or because relatives have 'given up' trying to influence the situation.
> *Collusion* includes those strategies where relatives actively

condone, support or collude with the behaviour. For example, with the negative symptoms, relatives may make undue 'allowance' for the illness and may indulge or reinforce social withdrawal. With delusions, on the other hand, relatives may 'go along' with the belief to avoid argument.

Reassurance is a strategy reported only in relation to positive symptoms where relatives present a calm, stable exterior, emphasising the security of the home and their relationship, but nevertheless not agreeing with the individual's beliefs or experiences.

Disorganised responses are those where relatives express feelings of desperation and helplessness, and engage in many strategies without consistency and without any clear dominant strategy emerging.

Constructive responses represent 'special action' taken by relatives to ameliorate the problem (but excluding coercive tactics).

The following examples show how some of these strategies relate to 'characteristic' problem behaviours.

Hallucinations and delusions

In one family Chris would frequently break off in mid-conversation and laugh inappropriately, and at other times he would shout out loud. His father would enquire about the content of the voices and would become dismissive and irritated by the interruptions:

> I would laugh at them to show him how stupid they are and I'd try to bring him to his senses and I'd say 'just watch the T.V., there's nothing going to happen' ('coercion').

In another family faced with a similar situation the individual's wife would collude with her husband and act as if she too heard the voices, to 'keep him company' ('collusion').

Relatives face a dilemma of whether to go along with the delusions, or to confront them directly. As indicated previously, attempts to challenge delusions rarely pay off, and relatives can end up irritated and dismissive of the individual's lack of 'reason'. Some relatives find a calmer, more detached approach helpful, in which they might empathise with the reality of the experience for the individual but firmly assert that it is not their own ('reassurance').

Negative or deficit behaviours

Families respond very differently to withdrawal and underactivity. In the Dawson family referred to above James spent much of his day alone in his room. His parents responded to this behaviour by taking his meals to his room and did not expect or encourage him to behave otherwise ('collusion'). Thus this family appear to condone James's behaviour but also in this case their strategy served to reduce their exposure to him due to their fear of his aggression ('avoidance').

In another family the relatives served meals only at certain times and expected basic domestic tasks to be undertaken by the individual and his brothers. They provided a basic structure to his day (which his parents prompted) and encouraged him to do things which he enjoyed prior to the illness onset (e.g. helping out at his father's working men's club) ('constructive').

Beyond the availability of specific coping behaviours, three themes recur in families which have some bearing on their coping efficacy. The first is the availability of alternatives. When first faced with schizophrenia some families quickly run into difficulty if they do not have the flexibility to try different approaches, and become entrenched. Families who respond to problems flexibly, trying out different approaches, seem to be among the most confident families with higher self-efficacy. This is clearly shown in the work of Falloon and colleagues, who have achieved considerable success with families, teaching them to develop and evaluate as many alternatives as possible before a course of action is undertaken (Falloon, Boyd, McGill, Razani, Moss and Gilderman, 1982). The second theme, however, is *consistency*. There is among some relatives a tendency to try everything at once (the 'disorganised' response) causing distress to themselves and confusion to the recipient. For similar reasons, consistency between family members is also important.

A third theme concerns the extent to which relatives feel they must 'make allowances' for behaviour which is the consequence of schizophrenia and, related to this, whether they perceive their role within a 'custodial' or a 'rehabilitative' framework. For example, in one instance a relative reported that as her son was receiving medication, and attending hospital as an outpatient, he therefore remained 'unwell' and felt it was her duty to care for him and not to make any undue demands on him. Those relatives who understand that there may be limits to the individual's abilities, and do not expect or aim to 'normalise' the behaviour, but who nevertheless set realistic standards, seem to fare better (see also Berkowitz, Kuipers,

Eberlein-Fries and Leff, 1981).

2. Concepts of schizophrenia

Myths

Perhaps the most common myth retained by relatives is that schizophrenics are inherently unpredictable and aggressive. The sense of intimidation and fear experienced by some relatives stems in part from this construction, which derives from split personality mythology and more recently from publicity given to the 'Yorkshire Ripper' case.

Illness vs. personality

Some relatives are inclined to view the behaviour of people with schizophrenia entirely within a personality framework. According to Vaughn (1977) this occurs predominantly in those families with a poor pre-illness relationship where personality constructions such as 'lazy' or 'selfish' continue to be used. Thus no distinction is made between behaviours which are directly related to schizophrenia (e.g. withdrawal) and those which are not. Clearly the effect of adopting such pernicious personality constructions impairs family relationships and can lead to punitive coping responses.

Symptoms and behaviour

Where relatives do not appreciate the relationship between the behaviour they observe and any associated psychotic phenomenology, unfortunate consequences can ensue. The parents of one quite disturbed individual were irritated and upset by his continued refusal to sit with them at mealtimes or to eat food prepared by them. Unbeknown to his parents, however, he was labouring under the delusion that his family were involved in a plot to kill him. In another case a mother's anger at her son's 'laziness' at his staying in bed all day was tempered by the knowledge that he believed he was receiving threatening 'messages' from the KGB about his neighbours and only felt safe in bed.

Expectations

The tenor of information gathered explicitly or implicitly from hospital staff about schizophrenia tends to be rather pessimistic or at the least very non-committal about the future, and about the role relatives can play (Creer and Wing, 1973). One relative remarked that he felt his

15

role was one of the 'orderly management of decline' and that 'all hope of a reasonable life together was gone'. His requests to the hospital for help were met with 'raised eyebrows and a shrug of the shoulders'. Clearly such low expectations can be self-fulfilling and destructive of coping efforts.

Maintenance medication

There is widespread misunderstanding about the function of maintenance medication among relatives and patients alike. In particular, the value of medication as a prophylactic is not well understood (Smith and Birchwood, 1987). This misunderstanding can lead to non-compliance because individuals are encouraged to take medication when relatively well (unlike many medications), and the benefits are not immediately apparent whereas the costs, in terms of side-effects, are. The experience of side-effects is the main cause of non-compliance (Hogan, Awad and Eastwood, 1983) and clearly education about the 'hidden' advantages of medication is crucial.

3. Family cohesion

The nature and effects of low family cohesion have already been discussed. Many families are, however, able to withhold the strain, and collectively can act in a positive therapeutic manner. Family cohesion may be considered to have two components. The first is a support function, being the degree of emotional proximity between key relatives and other non-affected family members. The second is a problem-solving function in which family members work together as a unit to define and resolve problems, including those arising within and without the family environment.

4. Communication

A number of research teams have identified families where conventional rules of adult communication and emotional proximity have been breached (Berkowitz *et al.*, 1981; Doane, Goldstein, Miklowitz and Falloon, 1986). In such families boundaries between the relative and the affected individual have broken down to such a degree that relatives are interacting in a manner more in keeping with a rather dependent and weak-willed child or adolescent. Relatives feel a need to talk and make decisions for the individual, who is credited with little initiative or responsibility. Take as an example the following extract from an interview by the authors with a relative and her 26-year-old daughter:

> she's not been doing well this week, she hasn't really tried at all, have you Sue? [looks to daughter shaking head] . . . she tried some baking as you suggested, I *gave* her all the ingredients and gave her all the help I could but she was so slow and kept on asking me what to do next so I just had to finish it off for her, didn't I Sue? [Question directed to S followed by pause] . . . come on Sue speak up . . . try and open your eyes . . . [Mother answers question] . . . Well, say goodbye Sue — you'll have to excuse her, she's forgotten her manners; just a bit shy today.

In this case, as in others, her mother feels her daughter needs close supervision and presents herself as a martyr to her daughter's cause.

Three characteristics summarise these relationships: poor communication skills (e.g. poor listening skills, making demands rather than requests); an over-protective management style (e.g. failure to encourage initiative) and the relatives' active sacrificing of their personal needs.

5. The neglect of personal and family needs

In addition to the neglect of personal needs of relatives which we referred to previously, the needs of other family members can be neglected; this may be of particular concern where there are young or adolescent siblings who may resort to acting out.

A thread running through these five dimensions of the family coping response is that essentially normal families are coping with disorder and are not primarily disordered themselves. This of course represents an apparent *volte-face* in the context of the long-held view that families represent the source of the pathogenesis in schizophrenia. Before attempting to integrate these elements of the family coping response and identify intervention possibilities, let us briefly examine the evidence from this alternative perspective to see what light is shed on family life in schizophrenia.

PROBLEM FAMILIES?

In this section the presence of abnormal family processes as a primary factor in the *psychogenesis* and *maintenance* of schizophrenia will be examined separately.

The rearing environment

Space precludes anything but a brief excursion into this important area, but the interested reader is directed to Hirsch and Leff's (1975) classic monograph on the subject. The subject at issue is whether the families of people with schizophrenia are *intrinsically* abnormal and pathogenic.

A number of theories have been proffered about the nature of these supposed 'schizophrenogenic' families, but the evidence for them is weak and contradictory and studies suffer from the problem that families are observed after the onset of schizophrenia, thus confounding cause and effect.

The Danish-American adoption studies bear directly on this issue (Kety, Rosenthal, Wender, Schulsinger and Jacobsen, 1975; Lowing, Mirsky and Pereira, 1983). These investigators identified individuals at high risk for schizophrenia (i.e. one or both biological parents were affected) who were adopted away within a month of birth into unaffected 'normal' families. These studies consistently show that the likelihood of developing schizophrenia among this 'high-risk' group does *not* vary in spite of quite profound changes in the rearing environment. The adoption technique is naturalistic and prone to bias; however at the very least the results show how difficult it is to break the cycle of schizophrenia from one generation to another through immersion of the high-risk individual in a 'normal' rearing environment, and thus that rearing by a schizophrenic parent is not a necessary (and certainly not a sufficient) condition for the emergence of schizophrenia. As this form of rearing has to be considered by family theorists as an extreme manifestation of 'schizophrenogenic' influences, then the basis for believing that the family has an independent role in the aetiology of schizophrenia must be seriously brought into question (Birchwood, Hallett and Preston, 1987).

Family life and the course of schizophrenia

In contrast, there is compelling evidence that family life can exert a considerable influence over the course and outcome of schizophrenia. This stems largely from the British studies of 'expressed emotion' (EE). Essentially, these studies have shown that relatives rated as 'high EE' (based mainly on critical comments made about the individual during his acute admission) were associated with a much higher rate of relapse in the individual in the 9 months after his discharge compared to those from 'low EE' families (58 vs 16 per cent). The study by Brown, Birley and Wing (1972) was replicated by Vaughn and Leff (1976), and when the samples were combined ($N=128$) an analysis revealed that EE, use of medication and duration of face-to-face contact between relative and patient, operated in a hierarchical, additive fashion. Thus individuals in *low* contact (less than 35 hours per week) with a high EE relative and taking regular medication showed a 15 per cent rate of relapse, comparable with the low EE group. Conversely, *high* contact with a high EE relative without the protective effect of medication predicted almost certain relapse (97 per cent).

The high EE measure clearly has a predictive value in its own right, and the functional equivalence of life events and high EE in precipitating relapse (Leff and Vaughn, 1980) supports the notion that high EE is an index of (chronic) stress in the family environment. However there must be doubt whether the EE concept itself can provide the means to develop the necessary descriptive and functional framework within which a model of the family interior can be developed if rational interventions are to follow. The EE concept is a typology and construes family characteristics as 'traits' in the same sense as personality or physical characteristics are individual traits. This trait construction is by its very nature an abstraction of family life which is potentially too rigid to accommodate its complexities. Thus, for example, it is unlikely that parents would be rated high EE in relation to all their offspring as the EE ratings are largely based on comments invited about schizophrenic symptoms and their development.

There is evidence from the original data reported by Brown *et al.* (1972), and Vaughn and Leff (1976), that high EE is not an endemic family trait but is a characteristic which *develops* with time. First of all, high EE tends to identify a more chronic group of individuals

Figure 2.1: The transactional' model

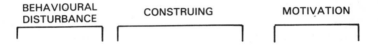

BEHAVIOURAL
DISTURBANCE   CONSTRUING   MOTIVATION

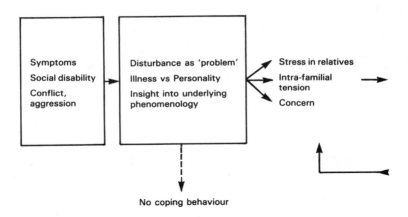

Symptoms	Disturbance as 'problem'	Stress in relatives
Social disability	Illness vs Personality	Intra-familial tension
Conflict, aggression	Insight into underlying phenomenology	Concern

No coping behaviour

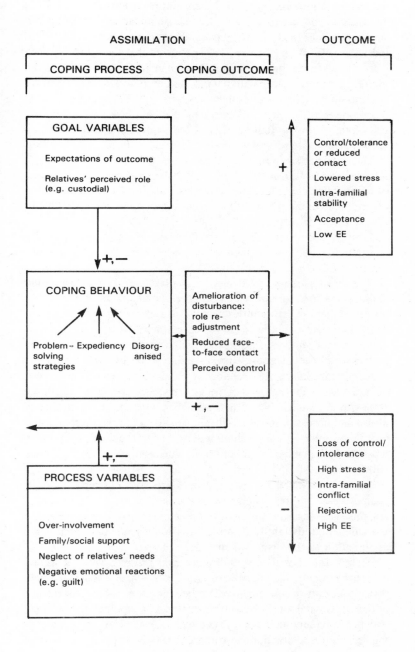

with more admissions ($\gamma = 0.51$), behavioural disturbance ($\gamma = 0.82$) and work impairment ($\gamma = 0.73$). Second, a comparison of the relationship between EE and relapse between first admission and readmitted individuals (Leff and Brown, 1977) showed that the effect is much weaker with first admissions: thus 38 per cent of first admissions from high EE families relapse within 9 months compared to 69 per cent for readmissions. This suggests that *with time* high EE families become more powerful in their influence, or that families are 'incorrectly classified' following first admission. Whichever is correct, it would seem that there are some developmental changes within these families.

One interpretation of these data is that families *emerge as high EE as chronicity advances*. This is not to deny the causal significance of family characteristics, but to suggest that high EE is a *visible* sign of pathological family disturbance which emerges as the outcome of a developmental process.

If this hypothesis is true, why should it be that some families emerge as high EE (i.e. change their behaviour toward the schizophrenic member) after a period of time?

The most parsimonious answer is that families differ in their abilities or efforts to *cope* with a disturbed family member: it has been observed that low EE families respond in a calmer fashion (Kuipers, 1979) but this has not been examined empirically, although there is evidence that families do differ in their coping styles, which bears a relationship to outcome (Birchwood, 1983). For most families, schizophrenia and its attendant behavioural anomalies will be a novel experience so there will not be an existing repertoire of coping strategies available on which to draw. These will have to be developed afresh and observations of families' adjustment to schizophrenia suggest that families do go through a period of trial and error in which the disturbed member is actively assimilated, but with varying results (Birchwood, 1983).

Under this model family influences are not construed as 'trait' characteristics in the systems theory sense, but as a learned coping response arising as a result of developmental interactions between the individual and his family ('transactions') whose primary goal is the assimilation of the disturbed member.

This 'transactional' model (Figure 2.1) presents what is argued to be the primary characteristic of families of schizophrenics, namely their propensity to assimilate a disturbed family member. A sequence of developmental interactions (transactions) is hypothesised between patient behaviour and the family coping response. The aim of the coping response is to ameliorate or improve relatives' perceived control over the disturbance or, if this fails, to reduce exposure to it. The outcome of this determines the affiliative quality of the relationship that ensues and the acceptance of the individual within the family system. The 'motor' of the assimilation process is the nature and severity of patient disturbance, the construing of this as a 'problem' and the ensuing stress, concern and intra-familial tension.

The assimilation process is facilitated (or restrained) by the operation of certain 'process' and 'goal' variables. Thus, for example, poor family cohesion or social support might dispose to a poor coping outcome through restricting the range of coping alternatives and heightening relatives' distress. A continuum of outcome is posited with the poles of the continuum as indicated in the figure. High EE may be synonymous with 'coping failure' and underpinned by certain kinds of (possibly coercive) coping strategies. Low EE occupies one section of the continuum and is associated with 'coping success' in terms of perceived control, low stress and successful familial assimilation. However, the means by which 'control', low EE and intrafamilial stability is achieved may not necessarily be through the deployment of exemplary coping strategies. In some instances relatives have, for example, sought to reinforce social withdrawal as a means of controlling their exposure to severe behavioural disturbance, thus preventing stressful confrontations (Birchwood, 1983).

FAMILY INTERVENTIONS: RESEARCH EVIDENCE

Three well-controlled family intervention studies have been undertaken in recent years, with very promising results.

The first such study of family intervention was conducted by Goldstein and his colleague in California (Goldstein and Kopeikin, 1981). Their intervention consisted of helping families identify stressful circumstances which might have precipitated the psychotic episode, to develop more effective stress-reducing strategies and to anticipate future ones. This was done to enable patients' return to the family environment, particularly with the first 6 weeks in mind, as they argue that this is the maximum risk period for relapse.

The intervention was structured as a sequence of four steps with later steps depending on the successful completion of earlier ones. The first step was largely educational, to highlight the role of stress in its onset and improve family cohesion. The first therapeutic objective was to arrive at concrete descriptions of two or three stressful situations within the family (e.g. arguments about the individual's

23

inactivity). The second step involved developing strategies for managing or avoiding these situations. The third step involved evaluating and refining these strategies. Finally, future difficulties were anticipated and planned for. Goldstein and Kopeikin reported a controlled trial over a 6-week post-discharge period varying drug level (average vs low) and family therapy in a 2 × 2 factorial design; 104 young people (mean age 23 years) with schizophrenia entered the trial and were randomly assigned to the groups.

The high dose/family therapy group showed a much lower rate of relapse compared to the low dose/no family therapy group at both 6 weeks (0 vs 24 per cent) and 6 months (0 vs 48 per cent). No differences emerged between the remaining groups. Goldstein reported significant effects of drug ($p<0.01$) and family therapy ($p<0.05$) over 6 months, but did not report the results of their interaction or data for all group comparisons. One is struck by the absence of relapse in the high dose/family therapy group and the ability of family therapy to halve the rate of relapse in the low dose treatment groups (48 vs 21 per cent) over 6 months. The study suggests that high dosage of medication and family intervention are functionally equivalent in forestalling relapse, and when both are present (or absent) an extreme of outcomes is obtained. This study suggests that the very early adjustment of families to schizophrenia (two-thirds were first-episode patients) may be crucial and a brief 6-week intervention can correct this before relatively permanent response characteristics set in. Thus the generalisability of this brief intervention to an older sample, and also the durability of its effects, remain uncertain.

The research team in London that were largely responsible for the renewed interest in family therapy as a result of their work on 'expressed emotion', reported the results of their intervention programme 4 years later (Leff, Kuipers, Berkowitz, Eberlein-Fries and Sturgeon, 1982).

Their study was a simpler comparison of two groups (both $N=12$) both stabilised on maintenance medication with one receiving the family intervention. In contrast to Goldstein their subjects were selected *a priori* as being at high risk of relapse (i.e. high contact with a 'high EE' family) and therefore were much older (35 vs 23 years). The intervention consisted of three components. The first was an educational package in which the relatives were informed about the nature, course and treatment of schizophrenia. The second was a relatives group in which high and low EE families met together and the therapists facilitated interactions between them. The rationale for this was that low EE families had found ways of coping with the everyday problems of living with schizophrenia, from which high EE families might learn. The third component of the intervention comprised individual sessions with families using 'dynamic interpretations or behavioural interventions'.

At 9 months follow-up there had been only one relapse (9 per cent) in the family intervention group compared with 50 per cent of the control group, although one of the intervention group was not available to follow up. This was maintained over 2 years (Leff, Kuipers, Berkowitz and Sturgeon, 1985) although this held only when patients who defaulted on medication were excluded from the analysis. The intervention led to a significant reduction in criticism which accounted for a reduction of EE in five of the eleven families, and in five families there was a reduction in face-to-face contact; overall the social intervention was successful in 73 per cent and in these families there was no relapse.

The appearance of the Leff et al. report was closely followed by a study undertaken by Ian Falloon and colleagues in California (Falloon et al., 1982). The Falloon intervention was highly structured and aimed to train individuals and families to recognise and resolve environmental stress within and outside the family. This was achieved by training families in a structured problem-solving technique and in interpersonal communication skills. They compared the family intervention ($N = 18$) with the best available individual community after-care ($N = 18$) including education about schizophrenia and vocational rehabilitative counselling. The contrast group therefore received an intensive psychosocial intervention. The subjects were some 10 years younger than Leff's, and most but not all came from high EE households.

Follow-up over 9 months showed a 6 per cent relapse rate in the family group (vs 44 per cent), matched by low readmission rate (11 vs 50 per cent) and lower monthly ratings of target symptoms. These results held up over 2 years of follow-up (Falloon, Boyd and McGill, 1984). Falloon also reports a greater tolerance of the families for social deficits, improved problem-solving effectiveness and improved family well-being. We are, however, not informed of any changes in EE. Falloon et al. found that the family intervention led to improved compliance with medication regimes; however, given maximum compliance the relapse rate is far lower than would be expected with drugs alone, and also the dosages of drugs required were much lower in the family group.

In two of the studies reviewed above the investigators did not restrict their sample to high EE families. This then raises a major question: is high EE sufficient to define all the important needs and risks associated with schizophrenia? This is unlikely. The index does appear to be a good short-term predictor of relapse. However, it remains to be seen whether these interventions can alter the course of schizophrenia in the long term, with or without longer-term family intervention. The prevention of short-term symptom exacerbation may turn out to be of only limited value in contrast to the individual's quality of life which these interventions generally have not emphasised. It is known from follow-up studies (e.g. Watt, Katz and Shepherd, 1983) that there are numerous individuals who are marginally maintained in the community with considerable psychiatric or social problems who are not regularly readmitted and who would be overlooked in the EE assessment procedure. It has also been suggested that low EE families may reduce relapse risk by reinforcing the individual's social withdrawal, thus alleviating stressful confrontations (Birchwood, 1983). Hence family interventions might be applied usefully to a broader range of individuals and their families than merely those who are high on EE. The important questions would then be within-group ones: what kinds of interventions help what kind of individual in what kind of family and with what kind of effect?

INTERVENTION STRATEGIES

Before considering the form which an intervention might take let us briefly bring together the specific needs which such an intervention might meet.

The needs of individuals with schizophrenia

1. Restitution of social and role functioning.
2. Prevention of relapse.
3. Reducing distress caused by persisting symptoms.
4. Amelioration of intra-familial relationship problems.

The needs of families

1. Information about schizophrenia, its symptoms and treatment, particularly as it applies to families' individual situations.
2. Amelioration of adverse family consequences including disturbed

family relationships, personal and social needs, financial/work difficulties and stress.

3. Amelioration of adverse emotional reactions in key relatives (e.g. guilt, stigma, embarrassment).

4. Practical advice on behavioural management and interaction skills.

Intervention procedures

On the basis of the transactional model outlined above, and the particular needs of patients and families, a three-stage intervention procedure is suggested. The primary function of the intervention is to assist families to improve their behavioural and emotional response to persisting behavioural disturbance in the affected family member in such a way as to meet the specific needs of the individual and his family. The following intervention model is perhaps somewhat different from existing or ongoing interventions in that it is entirely *needs-based* and does not rely on the EE measure as the primary index of need. The assessment of need — of the individual and his family — therefore forms an integral part of the overall intervention.

Assessment

Table 2.3 offers a basic set of assessments which may be used to assess 'need' for the individual and his family, and are currently used by the authors in Birmingham. The SBDS provides a detailed picture of disturbances, particularly those reported to be 'troublesome' by relatives. The social adjustment scales describe a profile of seven social functions including pro-social behaviour, recreations and independence. The family distress scale profiles the range of family hardships and consequences. The VCI provides a picture of family coping behaviour and the CFI and FIS provides a picture of family relationships including family cohesion, hostility and warmth.

Enabling family change

This second stage aims to overcome any constraints which have developed which will inhibit the coping efficacy of the family system. These constraints represent the 'construing', 'process' and 'goal' characteristics identified in the transactional model.

Understanding schizophrenia. Three areas of information might be covered. In the first, relatives should be provided with a general

Table 2.3: Some suggested assessment instruments

Characteristic	Measure
1. Schizophrenia	
Psychotic phenomenology	Present State Examination (PSE — Wing, Cooper and Sartorius, 1974)
Behavioural disturbance	Symptom-related Behavioural Disturbance (SBDS — Birchwood, 1983)
Social adjustment	Social Adjustment Scales (Birchwood, 1983)
2. Family	
Expressed emotion/ relapse risk	Camberwell Family Interview (CFI — Brown and Rutter, 1966)
Family burden/stress	Family Distress Scale — Extended (Pasamanick, Scarpitti and Dinitz, 1967); Symptom Rating Test (Kellner and Sheffield, 1973)
Coping behaviour	Video Coping Interview (VCI — Birchwood, 1983)
Family relationships	CFI/Family Interview Schedule (FIS — Birchwood, 1983)
Concepts of schizophrenia	Understanding Schizophrenia Scale (Smith and Birchwood, 1985)

orientation to the disorder. The notion of schizophrenia as a syndrome affecting thoughts, emotions and behaviour is offered. Specific myths may be discussed and questioned including that of split personality, inherent aggressiveness and the notion that families cause schizophrenia. Families frequently ask about the cause of schizophrenia and it may help to provide a basic summary of prevailing ideas.

The second area concerns the core symptoms. A simple description and examples of the major symptoms might be given; families find it helpful to learn how individuals experience these and first-hand accounts are helpful to improve empathy. Distinguishing between 'positive' and 'negative' symptoms is helpful as the latter are frequently construed in personality terms (e.g. 'laziness'), although the impression must not be conveyed that they are unmodifiable. The amelioration of negative symptoms through appropriate management should be stressed. Relatives should be taught how symptoms can translate into behaviour (e.g. voices leading to laughing and talking to self). Families should be provided with feedback about the symptoms present in their relative, how they affect his thinking and behaviour and influence relationships.

The third area covers the treatment of schizophrenia. The benefits, limitations and side effects of drugs should be outlined, emphasising the role of maintenance medication as a prophylactic.

It is helpful to back up information with written materials (e.g. Smith and Birchwood, 1985). The value of information provision has probably been underestimated. There is evidence that it can reduce stress, reduce personality constructions of 'schizophrenic' behaviour and increase family optimism (Berkowitz, Eberlein-Fries, Kuipers, and Leff, 1984). However, the *amount* of information which is assimilated is not as important as the *feeling* of being more knowledgeable (Smith and Birchwood, 1987).

Improving access and use of resources. Many families are isolated, or are at least not aware of the potential of familial and professional resources. Within the family, mention has already been made of the damaging effects of low family cohesion. The family's concern should be mobilised through involvement of family members in a collective therapeutic endeavour. The extended family can prove an invaluable resource if they are actively involved, and may serve to dilute the stress of managing severely disturbed individuals. Improving families' access to professional resources including day-care and recreational outlets can be helpful, as well as ensuring that families have a contact in emergencies. Providing families with information about disability benefits, tax allowances and the possibilities for longer-term support (e.g. hostels) may also be needed.

Amelioration of family hardship. One of the main tasks here is to ensure that relatives, and the family unit, do not neglect their own needs. Encouraging families to resume some leisure activities, by, for example, asking what they would otherwise be doing with their time, can be a useful tactic. Relatives may need encouragement and even targeting (i.e. direction) to achieve this; many are surprised that the 'catastrophes' which they imagine might take place if they leave the individual unattended rarely take place. Again those in very adverse situations should be encouraged to take 'breaks' away from home. Often resistance is encountered to these suggestions, usually because of guilt ('I am her mother and I am responsible for her welfare when she's ill, but I can't be a good mother if I spend an evening relaxing and enjoying myself'). Guilt can be reduced by pointing out to families that looking after their personal needs in this way can *improve* the

29

quality of their help through reducing stress on themselves. Meeting other families who have successfully accomplished this can be helpful.

Confronting negative emotions. The resolution of unhelpful emotions may derive from other components of the intervention, but in some cases they may need to be confronted directly. The first helpful step is to encourage relatives' insight into such emotions, how they relate to specific situations and inhibit change. For example, in one family the individual refused to come down from his room for meals. His mother took his meals to his room because otherwise she would feel guilty, particularly as her son would 'play on her emotions' about it. It was suggested that, by continuing to take his meals in this way, she was actually reinforcing his isolation; responding to her guilt may bring short-term relief to *her* but was of considerable long-term cost to her son. Coming face to face with her emotions, and their consequences for her and her son, enabled her to take the second but difficult step, which was to change her coping response to one of refusing to take his meals to him, which later led to his joining the family at mealtimes. In general, then, the sequence should be first to confront the emotions and their situational antecedents, to analyse their consequences for the individual and his relatives and to suggest an alternative coping response.

Improving family relationships. Mention has been made of situations where intra-familial boundaries have broken down to a degree where relatives are interacting in an over-protective and intrusive manner. Again relatives need to develop insight into their behaviour and its consequences in order to encourage change. This change can be brought about through instruction and communication skill training (Falloon *et al.*, 1984). These include training relatives: to listen in an 'active' way and to talk less in their interactions; to make requests rather than demands; to be explicit about their reasons for showing disapproval; and to encourage individuals to think and make decisions for themselves.

Managing schizophrenic disturbance

Interventions with families are clearly going to be time-limited, so it is important that the therapists do not act as a 'crutch', as this can lead to deterioration on termination of the major intervention. The provision of written materials should help here. More important, however, is the need for relatives to be taught to think and act independently, without the structure and prompting provided by the therapists.

The provision of a framework to facilitate such independence has been used with success by Ian Falloon and colleagues (Falloon *et al.*, 1982). These authors have adapted the problem-solving paradigm of D'Zurilla and Goldfried (1971), in which families are taught to clearly define the problem behaviour, to develop a range of possible solutions, to weigh the alternatives and to put into action their 'best' solution, over a reasonable period. This alone is often not sufficient for many families, who will initially need more direct guidance.

Two considerations must be weighed in the decision process. First of all, not all family-defined problems are problems for the individual with schizophrenia. In the case of the family who were embarrassed by their son's behaviour with their neighbour, the problem (embarrassment) was the family's — the neighbours may (or could) have been quite understanding. In other words the *legitimacy* of the problem should be first considered. Second, the solution to some problems may depend on an appreciation of relevant factors: for example, the individual who refuses medication may be unaware of its potential benefits; in a previous example the son's incessant provocation of his sister may be related to delusional beliefs and exacerbated by his sister's over-reaction.

Negative behaviours or deficits. A sequence of targets should be defined which are constructional in nature and build on areas of weakness. This can be done by employing detailed social adjustment scales. For example, in the case of a young man who spent all his time at home it was agreed to attempt to help him revive his former interest in gardening. This is best accomplished with the active participation and consent of the individual. Relatives need to be practised in the use of two component skills: the use of unobtrusive prompting (vs 'nagging') and encouraging relatives not to take for granted the individual's efforts, but to take time to consistently acknowledge appropriate behaviour. These techniques are often sufficient to create some movement which can then be built on. More formal 'contingency contracting' may be helpful in some cases to provide this initial change (see Case 2 below). This involves contracted agreement in which certain valued pay-offs are provided conditional on the completion of daily targets. Once some movement has been achieved this needs to be 'regularised' through engagement of support structures. This may include the use of sibling or extended family support, community resources, day units, social/recreation groups, employment rehabilitation centres, etc.

Case Example 1

Colin had a 2-year history of schizophrenia and remained actively hallucinated and deluded. He was out of work, withdrawn and very dependent on his mother. Following assessment it was decided to concentrate on his independence, recreational and pro-social skills. Colin enjoyed his food and he showed an interest in cooking. It was agreed that Colin would be given the opportunity to cook his favourite meals but that he had to learn to do so himself. His mother taught him basic cooking skills and he slowly accumulated a set of 'menu cards' with clearly labelled ingredients and step-by-step instructions. His sister helped him to shop and he learned how to budget using a calculator. After some weeks it was agreed that he should cook his own meals at weekends including the requisite shopping and budgeting. He was then prompted to resume his interest in gardening, fishing and the church. Eventually he structured his time using a timetable, and he attended a day centre 4 days a week. At present he and his family are engaged in converting part of his house to a flatlet, so that he can live semi-independently.

Case Example 2

Mark received a diagnosis of schizophrenia 9 months prior to his referral. He had no positive symptoms but was markedly inactive and listless. His only interest was his motorbike, which was in need of repair. Following a family round-table discussion about Mark's problems and his future, it was agreed that in exchange for his mother's financial (but now contingent) contribution towards his motorbike he agreed to undertake various domestic chores and to attempt to resume his social contacts.

He was later introduced to a Social Services day centre, to which he travelled on his motorbike. He found the activities useful but felt stigmatised. He was subsequently referred to an MSC employment rehabilitation centre, which provided him with useful work experience. He now works part-time in a wholesale market.

'Positive' behaviours. Severe positive symptoms can displace and impair pro-social behaviour and independence skills; similarly increasing pro-social and general activity levels can displace the acting out of psychotic thinking (Paul and Lentz, 1977). Thus among those who are severely disturbed, concentrating on developing assets will be of considerable benefit. However hallucinations, delusions and aggressive behaviours can be particularly disruptive of family life and

specific coping strategies will need to be developed in tandem with work on improving assets.

Family coping responses to hallucinations and delusions should be carefully examined to ensure that there is no tacit acknowledgement in the relatives' response of the veracity of the delusion. Some relatives become distressed and sometimes hostile when delusions are expressed. This should be discouraged, as this can only serve to destabilise the relationship. A strategy of 'constructive disengagement' should be urged, in which relatives are discouraged from lengthy discussion about their content, but to express understanding of the individual's views and to state firmly that they are not their own.

Disconfirmation can sometimes be suggested with focal encapsulated delusions (e.g. one mother sampled the glass of wine she poured for her son who suddenly believed his parents had poisoned it). On the other hand, if the delusion is a part of a wider delusional system, 'special action' of this sort can raise rather than quell suspicion.

Aggressive behaviour is perhaps the most difficult to help families to cope with. Once the family has acquiesced to any form of intimidation or anti-social conduct, it becomes difficult for families to restore control. If possible families should be urged to set clear limits and to clearly define what is acceptable. Families should avoid responding with aggression as this can establish an undesirable *modus operandi*. Sanctions should be made explicit, and in cases of repeated physical assault the assistance of the police should be raised as a possibility. The prevention of aggression is clearly the best approach, and an attempt should be made to establish any function the aggression may have (e.g. in the Dawson family James's aggressive conduct seemed to be directed at the weakest link and cause maximum disruption).

Case Example 1

Keith's wife had a 5-year history of schizophrenia. A recurring theme in her thinking was that Keith exerts a form of control over her through the things he says and in the way he touches her hair. She has also accused him of infidelity. Keith was extremely distressed by her behaviour and would experience severe disappointment if, as often happened, she would go for 2 or 3 days without any accusations then 'relapse'. He would become very involved with the vicissitudes of her thinking and would discuss her delusions at length with her. It was suggested to Keith that his admonitions would not significantly change her beliefs, and

33

that he was unnecessarily distressing himself, which was probably making his wife insecure and unstable. It was suggested that he should disengage himself from his wife's delusions, firmly assert his point of view without being patronising, be calm and unmoved and desist from extensive discussion about them. They were urged to take various practical steps to improve their life together, such as going out regularly, finding new outlets, etc. Keith found a dramatic improvement in their relationshp in spite of her delusions and was much less tearful and stressed.

Case Example 2

Mr and Mrs Davies's son Elliot had taken to smoking marijuana since the onset of schizophrenia. He spent a lot of his time in his room smoking and would do very little for himself. His parents had attempted to get him to take on some responsibility for himself but Elliot threatened his parents and on many occasions assaulted his father. The parents felt helpless and were afraid for their safety. At a case conference in a day unit attended by Elliot and his parents, the parents agreed that unless Elliot stopped smoking, and tried to do more things for himself, he would not be welcome at home, and that a short-term place would be made available at the hospital if he wished. It was indicated to Elliot that the police would be called if there were any further assaults. Elliot stopped smoking at home but his parents were unable to motivate him. He was finally found a place at a hostel with a highly structured self-help regime. He started to go home on weekend leave and his parents were trained to continue his programme and to improve their interaction style with Elliot. He spends increasing time at home. There have been no further aggressive incidents.

CONCLUSION: SERVICE CONSIDERATIONS

It remains an open question whether interventions with families can alter the course of schizophrenia. Research questions have necessarily been rather crude and based on small samples. There is little in the way of theory to guide and operationalise family interventions, and hitherto interventions have assumed a uniformity of needs between families and a uniformity of intervention with individuals diagnosed 'schizophrenic'. Research should ultimately be able to answer the question: 'What kind of intervention is appropriate with what kind of individual in what kind of family and with what kind of effect?'

It is unlikely (but not proven) that family interventions will ever replace the need for neuroleptic drugs, but there is evidence that, within limits, they can act as mutual substitutes, but that the best outcome is seen with a combination of both.

Whatever the ultimate outcome of this research may be, the needs of families that it has brought to wider attention and their crucial role in community maintenance will remain. There is now sufficient understanding of these families, their needs and intervention possibilities to consider the provision of routine services to this group.

There will be scepticism about the concept of a service to families because of the widespread assumption that families are potentially 'pathological' (which family intervention aims to correct). What has been stressed in this chapter is that families themselves have genuine needs which should not be overlooked, in addition to their being in an ideal position to favourably influence the individual's quality of life. For these reasons, families should be construed not as possible impediments but as *partners* in the overall management of schizophrenia. Indeed this is a role which self-help groups such as the National Schizophrenia Fellowship have long advocated.

A successful alliance between the family and the psychiatric service cannot be undertaken on a low-cost, piecemeal, unplanned basis. The interventions outlined in this chapter require close integration with conventional psychiatric management. This in turn requires managerial support in terms of policy (especially that of rehabilitation), finance and professional resources.

One service model is currently being evaluated in the West Birmingham Health Authority by the authors in conjunction with Raymond Cochrane (University of Birmingham). This authority has funded a family service run by clinical psychologists and support staff. The 'Family Centre for Advice, Resources and Education' offers interventions of the kind outlined here to all appropriate individuals with acute schizophrenia during and after their hospital stay. The service also offers short education courses and intensive interventions to families where the individual is not immediately subject to acute admission. A further aspect of this partnership which is under study attempts to train families to recognise and measure early signs of schizophrenic relapse and, through the Centre, to alert the medical team to ensure a prompt increase in maintenance medication to a therapeutic level in order to forestall relapse. The Service is viewed as an integral part of the overall management of individuals with schizophrenia, and maintains a variety of close links with community resources, including the National Schizophrenia Fellowship, Social Services, voluntary groups and the local Health Promotion Unit. Research over the past 10 years has raised expectations among people with schizophrenia, their families, and not least psychiatric professionals. Let us hope that future services are planned which can properly translate theory into practice.

REFERENCES

Berkowitz, R., Kuipers, L. Eberlein-Fries, R. and Leff, J. (1981) Lowering expressed emotion in relatives of schizophrenics. In M. Goldstein (ed.), *New directions for mental health services: 12 New developments in interventions with families of schizophrenics*, Jossey-Bass, San Francisco, pp. 27–46

Berkowitz, R., Eberlein-Fries, R., Kuipers, L. and Leff, J. (1984) Educating relatives about schizophrenia, *Schizophrenia Bulletin, 10*, 418–29

Birchwood, M.J. (1983) Family coping behaviour and the course of schizophrenia: a two year follow-up study. Unpublished PhD thesis, University of Birmingham

Birchwood, M.J., Hallett, S.E. and Preston, M.C. (1987) *Schizophrenia: an integrated approach to research and treatment*, Longman Applied Psychology Series, London

Brown, G.W. and Rutter, M.L. (1966) The measurement of family activities and relationships, *Human Relations, 19*, 241–63

Brown, G.W., Birley, J.L.T. and Wing, J.K (1972) The influence of family life on the course of schizophrenic disorders: a replication, *British Journal of Psychiatry, 121*, 241–58

Creer, C. and Wing, J.K. (1973) *Schizophrenia in the home*, National Schizophrenia Fellowship, Surbiton, Surrey

Doane, J.A., Goldstein, M.J., Miklowitz, D.J. and Falloon, I.R.H. (1986) The impact of individual and family treatment on the affective climate of families of schizophrenics, *British Journal of Psychiatry, 148*, 279–87

D'Zurilla, T.J. and Goldfried, M.R. (1971) Problem solving and behaviour modification, *Journal of Abnormal Psychology, 78*, 107–26

Falloon, I.R.H., Boyd, J.L., McGill, C.W., Razani, J., Moss, H.B. and Gilderman, A.M. (1982) Family management in the prevention or exacerbation of schizophrenia: a controlled study, *New England Journal of Medicine, 306*, 1437–40

Falloon, I.R.H., Boyd, J.L. and McGill, C.W. (1984) *Family care of schizophrenia: a problem solving approach to the treatment of schizophrenia*, Guilford Press, New York

Gibbons, J.S., Horn, S.H., Powell, J.M. and Gibbons, J.L. (1984) Schizophrenic patients and their families: a survey in a psychiatric service based on a DGH unit, *British Journal of Psychiatry, 144*, 70–7

Goldman, H. (1980) The post-hospital mental patient and family therapy: prospects and populations, *Journal of Marital and Family Therapy, 6*, 447–52

Goldstein, M.J. and Kopeikin, H.S. (1981) Short and long term effects of

36

combining drug and family therapy. In M.J. Goldstein (ed.), *New directions for mental health services: 12 New developments in interventions with families of schizophrenics.* Jossey-Bass, San Francisco, pp. 5–26

Hewitt, K.E. (1983) The behaviour of schizophrenic day-patients at home: an assessment by relatives, *Psychological Medicine, 13,* 885–9

Hirsch, S.R. and Leff, J.P. (1975) *Abnormalities in parents of schizophrenics,* Maudsley Monograph 22, Oxford University Press, London

Hogan, T.P., Awad, A.G. and Eastwood, R. (1983) A self-report scale predictive of drug compliance in schizophrenics: reliability and discriminative validity, *Psychological Medicine, 13,* 177–83

Kellner, R. and Sheffield, B.F. (1973) A self-rating scale of distress, *Psychological Medicine, 3,* 88–100

Kety, S.S., Rosenthal, D., Wender, P.H., Schulsinger F. and Jacobsen, B. (1975) Mental illness in the biological and adoptive families of adoptive individuals who have become schizophrenic: a preliminary report based on psychiatric interviews. In R.R. Fieve, D. Rosenthal, and H. Brill (eds), *Genetic research in psychiatry,* Johns Hopkins University Press, Baltimore, pp. 45–71

Kint, M.G. (1977) Problems for families versus problem families, *Schizophrenia Bulletin, 3,* 355–6

Kuipers, L. (1979) Expressed emotion: a review, *British Journal of Social and Clinical Psychology, 18,* 237–43

Leff, J.P. and Brown, G.W. (1977) Family and social factors in the course of schizophrenia (letter), *British Journal of Psychiatry, 130,* 417–20

Leff, J.P. and Vaughn, C.E. (1980) The interaction of life events and relatives' expressed emotion in schizophrenia and depressive neurosis, *British Journal of Psychiatry, 136,* 146–53

Leff, J.P., Kuipers, L., Berkowitz, R., Eberlein-Fries, R. and Sturgeon, D. (1982) A controlled trial of social intervention in families of schizophrenic patients, *British Journal of Psychiatry, 141,* 121–34

Leff, J.P., Kuipers, L., Berkowitz, R. and Sturgeon, D. (1985) A controlled trial of social intervention in the families of schizophrenic patients: 2 year follow up, *British Journal of Psychiatry, 146,* 594–600

Lowing, P.A., Mirsky, A.F. and Pereira, R. (1983) The inheritance of schizophrenia spectrum disorders: a reanalysis of the Danish adoptee study data, *American Journal of Psychiatry, 140,* 1167–71

Pasamanick, B., Scarpitti, F. and Dinitz, S. (1967) *Schizophrenics in the community,* Appleton-Century-Crofts, New York

Paul, G.L. and Lentz, R.J. (1977) *Psychological treatment of chronic mental patients: milieu vs. social learning programmes,* Harvard University Press, Cambridge, Mass.

Smith, J.V.E. and Birchwood, M.J. (1985) *Understanding Schizophrenia 1–4,* West Birmingham Health Promotion Unit, Health Education Council

Smith, J.V.E. and Birchwood, M.J. (1987) Specific and non-specific effects of educational interventions with families of schizophrenic patients, *British Journal of Psychiatry* (in press)

Vaughn, C.E. (1977) Patterns of interaction in families of schizophrenics. In H. Katschanig (ed.), *Schizophrenia: the other side,* Urban and Schwartzeberg, Vienna, pp. 105–21

Vaughn, C.E. and Leff, J.P. (1976) The influence of family and social factors on the course of psychiatric illness: a comparison of schizophrenic and depressed neurotic patients, *British Journal of Psychiatry, 129,* 125–37

Watt, D.C., Katz, K. and Shepherd, M. (1983) The natural history of schizophrenia: a 5-year prospective follow-up of a representative sample of schizophrenics by means of a standardised clinical and social assessment, *Psychological Medicine,* 13, 603–70

Wing, J.K., Cooper, J.E. and Sartorius, N. (1974) *The measurement and classification of psychiatric symptoms,* Cambridge University Press, London

3

Families with Mentally Handicapped Children

Jan Pahl and Lyn Quine

The birth of a mentally handicapped child does not necessarily imply, in the words of the title of this book, that there will be disorder in the family. It is important to begin by stressing that the skills and abilities of the children with whom we are concerned are very varied. Some are seriously intellectually impaired, immobile and incontinent, while others are able to read, write and count. The behaviour of some children is such that they can never be taken into a public place without fear of embarrassment, while others are cheerful, easy-going people who make friends wherever they go. There has been much debate about the appropriate term to use in describing this very varied group of children. The phrase 'mentally retarded' has given way, in Britain at least, to 'mentally handicapped', which is itself being replaced by 'children with severe learning difficulties'. This last phrase reminds us that these are first and foremost children, but children whose intellectual capacities are impaired.

There is a long-standing debate about the extent to which a family containing a handicapped child is likely to be a handicapped family. This debate is often presented in terms of a contrast between a 'pathological' and a 'normal' model of the family (Wilkin, 1979; Tew, Payne and Laurence, 1974). Studies which adopt the first model have devoted much effort to scoring the amount of guilt and shame, rejection and over-protection shown by parents of handicapped children. The pathological model still underlies much professional thinking about the care, treatment and support of mentally handicapped people and their families. On the one hand parents who adapt family life to cope with the child's impairments may be accused of being 'over-protective', while those who try to maintain normal patterns of family life may be accused of 'failing to accept' the child's handicap. Parents who demand more short-term care for their child may be seen as 'rejecting', while those who refuse offers of short-term care may be defined as 'over-anxious'. By contrast with the pathological model, the second approach emphasises the essential normality of these families. As Wilkin says:

> Where the normal family model is used, the fact that problems are experienced by the family is not denied, but the assumption that one should always look for harmful effects is questioned. (Wilkin, 1979, p. 33)

There is no doubt that the birth of a handicapped child can have profound effects on a family, but it is not necessarily accurate to see these effects in terms of 'disorder'.

There are problems, too, about the use of the term 'family'. The idea of the family as a social group consisting of an earning husband, a wife who is responsible for domestic work and their dependent children is increasingly anachronistic. In Britain in 1983 over half of all married women were in paid employment, 13 per cent of families were headed by a single parent, and families with one breadwinner were rarer than families with two or no breadwinners. Families with an earning husband, a dependent wife and two children composed a mere 5 per cent of all households (Study Commission on the Family, 1983). Thus it would be more accurate to replace the term 'the family' with 'families', and to recognise that, while some forms of the family typically face greater difficulties than others, the many different forms of the family all reflect individual choices about the ways people prefer to live (Barrett and McIntosh, 1982; Close and Collins, 1985).

This chapter will be concerned mainly with severely mentally handicapped children, who are defined as those whose IQs are around or below 50 and whose intellectual abilities are seriously impaired. Traditionally they are distinguished from the mildly mentally handicapped, who have IQs of between 50 and 70: however, recognition of the arbitrary nature of these classifications has led to an increasing reluctance to categorise children by IQ. It is estimated that between four and five children out of every thousand are likely to be severely mentally handicapped, and of these over 90 per cent live at home with their parents (Mittler, 1979a). What does the birth of a mentally handicapped child mean to a family? Is the child likely to be a source of stress, and, if so, which impairments are most stressful for parents? What is the impact on the parents' marriage and on the siblings? What aids and services do families find most helpful? This chapter will consider these and other questions; we shall draw evidence from a number of different studies, but the main source will be our own research into the needs of families with handicapped children (Pahl and Quine, 1984).

THE STUDY OF FAMILIES WITH SEVERELY MENTALLY HANDICAPPED CHILDREN

The aim of our study was to investigate the stresses involved in caring for a mentally handicapped child at home, and to assess the extent to which different services were able to relieve the burden on families. The research was funded by the South East Thames Regional Health Authority, the Medway Health Authority and the South East Kent Health Authority. The study had two main stages, which we have called the 'population survey' and the 'sample survey'. The first stage involved assessing the total population of severely mentally handicapped children aged 0-16 in two health districts, using the Disability Assessment Schedule developed by Holmes, Shah and Wing (1982). The second and main stage of the study involved interviews with a sample of 200 families, selected from the 399 whose children had been assessed in the population survey. A stratified random sample of 100 families was selected from one health district and these were matched with 100 families from the other health district so that the study should have a quasi-experimental design. Structured questionnaires were used to interview the people who were responsible for the day-to-day care of the children: 190 of the carers were the natural mothers and the rest included foster parents, grandparents and one father. This chapter presents selected data from the study, setting this in a broader context by drawing on other studies of families with mentally handicapped children.

What impairments affected the children in our study? In the population survey the assessments collected information about mobility, continence, self-help skills, behaviour, medical and psychiatric conditions and sensory impairments. Table 3.1 sets out the main problems which the children faced, and shows how our population compared with a much larger, national sample of children surveyed in a study carried out for the Jay Committee (DHSS, 1979). The Jay Report made a distinction between children living in hospitals and those in hostels, and Table 3.1 shows that in many respects the children in our study were more akin to the hospital population. For example, about a third of the children in our study were unable to walk by themselves, a proportion similar to that for the hospital children and

41

far higher than that for the hostel children. In a variety of other ways the children in our study were much more impaired than the mentally handicapped children which the Jay Committee found living in residential hostels. Two-thirds of our children were unable to wash and dress themselves, nearly half had some sort of behaviour problem, a third were doubly incontinent, a third suffered from epileptic fits, a fifth were blind or partially sighted, and an eighth had hearing difficulties. Twenty years ago many of these children would have been offered residential care, probably in a hospital, and their parents would have been urged to relinquish them, both for the sake of the rest of the family, and for the sake of the children themselves. Now, with the tide flowing in favour of community care, these children are remaining at home. The interviews showed what this meant for these families and for those who are responsible for the day-to-day care of severely handicapped children.

Table 3.1: Disabilities of mentally handicapped children

	Jay Report (DHSS, 1979)		Pahl/Quine Study
	Hospital units and wards (%)	Residential homes (%)	Children at home (%)
Unable to walk by themselves	34	8	34
Unable to feed without help	51	24	43
Unable to wash and dress themselves	79	44	68
Severe behaviour problems	50	34	42
Doubly incontinent during the day	55	15	33
Blind or partially sighted	11	4	19
Deaf and could not use hearing aid	5	3	13
Epilepsy (including controlled epileptics)	44	18	30
N	673	325	399

The effect on family living standards

The interviews with the 200 parents in the sample showed that the presence of a severely mentally handicapped child affected families in a variety of different ways. The employment pattern in these households differed from that which might have been expected in a sample of families with growing children. These differences mainly affected the mothers, of whom only 5 per cent were in full-time employment and 21 per cent in part-time employment. This was at a time when in Britain as a whole 17 per cent of women with children under 16 were in full-time employment and 35 per cent were in part-time employment (Martin and Roberts, 1984, p. 13). This means that the employment rate for mothers with a handicapped child is exactly half the rate of that for mothers whose children are not mentally handicapped. Of those mothers who were not in employment, half would have liked paid work; the majority of these said that they were prevented from taking a job by their responsibility for the handicapped child. As far as fathers were concerned, 83 per cent were in full-time employment, 13 per cent were unemployed and the remainder were either retired or disabled. This was at a time when the unemployment rate in South East England was 9.5 per cent, so there was a rather higher rate among the men in our sample, by comparison with the general population.

A number of other studies have explored the financial impact of caring for a mentally handicapped child at home (see, for example, Baldwin, 1985; Buckle, 1984; Townsend, 1979). Our data on housing, on consumer goods, and on income all support the findings of other research that having a handicapped child penalises families financially in a number of different ways. Firstly, the responsibility for the care of the child tends to reduce family income, particularly by making it difficult for mothers to earn, but also by limiting fathers' ability to do overtime. Of those mothers who did earn, 30 per cent said that their role as carers caused a reduction in earnings. Among employed fathers, 35 per cent said that loss of overtime or shift work reduced their earnings, while 20 per cent of unemployed fathers said that responsibility for the handicapped child reduced their capacity to work.

Secondly, the needs of the handicapped child meant extra expenditure on items such as clothing, bedding, footwear, and on washing and drying. Keeping immobile or sick children warm implies heavy heating bills. Incontinence and dribbling may result in heavy wear on clothes, as does constant rocking, pulling or rubbing. Footwear may be worn unevenly by a partly mobile or hyperactive child. Clothes or shoes may have to be specially made. Here are some of the comments parents made:

She has to have her shoes made specially. These cost £120. They were paid for by a charity. I don't know what we'll do when they wear out.

43

> I spend more on clothes than for the others, partly to get a good fit, but mainly because I think it is important that she looks really good. It helps me when I take her out, if she is complimented, and it makes her more acceptable to other people.

> He tears all his clothes. I can't put him in anything constricting because he tears it straight off.

> She dribbles all the time, and after a while it sort of stains all her jumpers. I like her to look nice because I think it compensates.

> We get through ever such a lot of sheets. They have to be washed every day because he's doubly incontinent, and they wear out.

Thirdly, as a consequence of their lower incomes and greater financial responsibilites, families had to cut back in other areas. The proportions who owned cars, or who had central heating, were lower than national figures for ownership of these goods in households with children. Many of the families were worried about money: for a quarter of the families whom we interviewed money was a constant worry, while altogether 58 per cent had some anxiety about being able to cope financially.

Who does the work involved in caring?

The work of caring for a severely handicapped child has been described as 'the daily grind of care' (Bayley, 1973). Glendinning said:

> The day-to-day care needed by a severely disabled child in many respects represents a prolonging of the dependencies of early childhood long past the ages at which they would normally cease. Thus the bathing, feeding, toileting, lifting and carrying, continuous attention and supervision, disturbed sleep and restricted social life which are common features of looking after an infant can persist for many years and, indeed, can become increasingly difficult as the child gets heavier and the parents grow older. (Glendinning, 1983, p. 41)

A number of studies have shown that it is normally the mother who shoulders this burden (Bayley, 1973; Hewett, Newson and Newson, 1970; Parker, 1985; Wilkin, 1979; Younghusband, Birchall, Davie and Kellmer-Pringle, 1970). In our study we were interested to know whether this pattern still continued, and whether, at a time of high unemployment, fathers without paid work did more of the work of caring. Respondents were asked whether their partners helped with child care 'every day', 'most days', 'once or twice a week', 'less often' or 'never'. In all cases where this question was appropriate the respondent was a woman living with her husband.

The number of husbands who helped every day was very small. The tasks which husbands were most likely to perform were lifting and carrying the child, but only a third of husbands whose child required lifting and carrying did this every day. For all the other tasks involved in the care of a handicapped child the numbers helping every day were much smaller. The percentages were based on the totals of those children whose care required that the task be done: we did not ask if a father changed nappies if the child was continent. The percentages of fathers who helped on a daily basis were as follows: feeding the child, 18 per cent; changing nappies, 15 per cent; toileting, 12 per cent; getting up in the night, 11 per cent; dressing and washing the child, 10 per cent.

When we looked at fathers who helped once or twice a week the numbers involved were somewhat larger, though it must be remembered that in some cases the help provided by these fathers represented a very small proportion of the work that had to be done. There were no significant differences between the social classes in terms of the amount of work which fathers did, but unemployed fathers were more likely to help than were employed fathers. This reflects partly the fact that unemployed fathers are likely to be at home during the day, and partly the recognition by some fathers that their help was badly needed. Thus the mother of a multiply handicapped 10-year-old, who suffered from cerebral palsy, said, 'We only just get by. Both of us spend all the time looking after Bob. In fact, I don't know how I'd manage if my husband got a job.'

Alternative sources of help might be the siblings of the handicapped child and the friends, neighbours and relations of the family. How much help did the chief carers get from these sources? Out of the total sample, 151 families had other children over 5, and these respondents were asked whether their children helped with the care of the handicapped child or with housework. The results showed that less than 10 per cent of the siblings carried out domestic tasks alone, 22 per cent sometimes helped the mother with the handicapped child and 28 per cent helped with housework. Thus, though siblings do help, they provide even less support to carers than do husbands. Our results are rather similar to those of Wilkin, who concluded:

Whether or not children provided assistance was related to their age and sex. . . . Support rose to a peak in the 12-16 age group where three quarters provided some assistance and almost a third had a high level of participation. Among the 16+ age group the level of support dropped sharply as children found jobs and left home. Thus the greatest potential for support seems to be among the 12-16 group, but within this group it is quite heavily concentrated among girls. This difference between the contribution to the domestic routine of girls and boys suggests that the sexual division of labour in parental roles is in the process of being repeated in the next generation. (Wilkin, 1979, p. 137)

The point about the help provided by teenage sisters, and a few brothers, is important for those concerned with what happens to handicapped children when they reach adulthood. Policies for community care suggest that the ideal is that mentally handicapped adults should be able to live, like other citizens, in ordinary houses in the community. However, unless there is a very large expansion of provision for mentally handicapped people, it is likely that many will simply continue to live at home with their parents. As the other children of the family leave home these parents will have to take on an increasing burden of care.

Community care policies also stress the importance of help from outside the immediate family. For example, the 1971 White Paper, in its general principles, stated that:

Understanding and help from friends and neighbours and from the community at large are needed to help the family to maintain a normal social life and to give the handicapped member as nearly a normal life as his handicap or handicaps permit. (DHSS, 1971, p. 10)

How much help do families actually get from friends, neighbours and relations? Table 3.2 shows the extent to which the families we interviewed could count on receiving help on a day-to-day basis. The only significant type of help given by people outside the immediate family was moral support. By comparison, little practical help was received with child care and household tasks. Though many mothers said that they valued the moral support they received, it was clear that people outside the family did little to lighten the burden of care.

The picture that we found was very similar to that described by Wilkin, who used a detailed questionnaire to document exactly how

Table 3.2: Families who received help from relatives, friends and neighbours

	Sources of help					
	Wife's family		Husband's family		Friends and neighbours	
Help with	Help most days (%)	Occa-sional help (%)	Help most days (%)	Occa-sional help (%)	Help most days (%)	Occa-sional help (%)
Baby-sitting	4	37	3	23	4	35
Housework	4	9	2	4	0	5
Taking children	5	21	2	11	1	17
Shopping/transport	3	15	2	7	1	15
Moral support	25	28	14	13	25	20

much help of different types was received from various different sources. Wilkin concluded:

> The term community care for a mentally handicapped child refers to care *in* the community and not care *by* the community. The nuclear family is the framework in which the child is cared for. Within the family it is mothers who carry the major burden of care usually with relatively little support from other family members. The contribution of people outside the family to the practical burden of care is almost negligible. (Wilkin, 1979, p. 146)

Social isolation

One effect of lack of support from friends and neighbours is that parents feel themselves to be socially isolated. In our study many parents had difficulties in finding a baby-sitter if they wanted to go out, and some never went out in the evening unless they took the handicapped child with them. Altogether 52 per cent of the mothers said that having a handicapped child prevented them from going out as frequently as they would have liked. In answer to the question 'Some people say that having a handicapped child makes a mother very lonely; do you think this is true from your experience?', 45 per cent of respondents said 'yes'. Mothers who said the child prevented them from going out, or who felt lonely because of the presence of the child, were significantly more likely to be stressed, as assessed by the

Malaise Inventory, which we describe below. Some mothers spoke of the embarrassment which people felt in the presence of the handicapped child, and described how this led to problems in making and maintaining relationships. One said: 'I feel like an outsider — I don't feel the same as everyone else — I have nothing in common with them.' The mother of a severely handicapped and behaviourally disordered teenager said: 'Geoffrey's problems are too embarrassing for someone else to cope with. His anti-social behaviour is difficult. Also cleaning him up after he has wet and dirtied himself is not something anyone else could be asked to do.' Some parents expressed an alternative view. One said: 'I have made friends through her — people from church show a special interest in her.'

However, in general the presence of the handicapped child, especially if he or she had behaviour problems, had the effect of cutting the parents off from others. This social isolation could extend to the mentally handicapped child and to other members of the family. Many of the handicapped children had no relationships with children outside the family, apart from those they met at school. Over half never went out to play with other children or had others in to play with them.

Effects on the siblings and on the marriage

Previous studies have suggested that having a handicapped child may present serious problems of adjustment to the family (Tizard and Grad, 1961). Some have suggested that the mental health of siblings may be affected. Gath, for example, measured psychiatric disorder in the siblings of Down's syndrome children by means of behaviour ratings made by parents and teachers. She found significantly more psychiatric disorder in these children by comparison with the siblings of normal children, with a particularly marked increase in psychiatric disorder among girls with handicapped siblings (Gath, 1978).

In our study, parents were ambivalent about the effects on brothers and sisters of having a handicapped sibling. Asked whether the other children had benefited at all, three-quarters agreed that there had been gains; however, about half the parents saw the difficulties surrounding the handicapped child as a disadvantage to the family. Some parents were concerned that the other children would suffer, for example, because the handicapped child disturbed their activities or because they felt inhibited about asking friends home; other parents suggested that the presence of the handicapped child had made the other children kinder and more tolerant. The sample were fairly evenly divided on this point, about half feeling that coping with handicap had been a disadvantage and a restriction to the family, while the other half felt it had not made much difference. Asked whether the overall impact on the family had been adverse, 44 per cent said 'yes', 42 per cent 'no' and 14 per cent were unsure.

When parents spoke of the effects on the other children the behaviour of the handicapped child was clearly important. Many made comments like these:

He makes them appreciate good health — value life — live each day as it comes. It makes them less selfish.

It's made them more understanding towards handicapped people and their problems, and more sympathetic.

But when the child was not only handicapped but also had severe behaviour problems, the parents were likely to see the effects on their other children as harmful:

He affects their sleeping and dominates the house. They need protection from him as he is violently aggressive. The girls especially are physically hurt by him.

The other children have had such a bad experience that they resent handicap — have nothing to do with it. We've lost contact with them to some extent.

Emotionally and socially it has affected them. The sexual problem affects the girls — their friends' parents have to keep an eye on what is happening between them. The oldest girl is unwilling to stay in the house alone with James.

Having a handicapped child can also have important implications for the parents' marriage. We have explored this issue more fully elsewhere, and have demonstrated that the stress of caring for a mentally handicapped child can be mitigated by a good marriage or by a husband who gives real help with the work of caring for the child (Quine and Pahl, 1987). Other research has shown the importance of a close and confiding relationship in reducing the likelihood of depression in women (Brown and Harris, 1978). In our study of families with handicapped children we found that mothers who had someone in whom they could confide were less likely to be stressed than those who lacked such a relationship. Additionally, having a mentally handicapped child did seem to be associated with feelings of social isolation, both for the carer and for other members of the family.

The stress of caring for a mentally handicapped child

We have shown that mentally handicapped children have a variety of different impairments and that they can create a variety of problems for the families into which they are born. In this section we shall investigate exactly what it is about having a mentally handicapped child which is most stressful for the carer. Is a very dependent child necessarily a greater burden than a less dependent child? Are children with Down's syndrome really easier to care for? How stressful is difficult behaviour compared with incontinence or immobility? How much do financial worries, extra work and social isolation add to the stress of caring? In answering these questions we shall be summarising arguments which we have developed at greater length elsewhere (see especially Pahl and Quine, 1984; Quine and Pahl, 1985). A large body of literature has claimed that mothers of handicapped children are vulnerable to stress (see, for example, Bradshaw and Lawton, 1978; Glendinning, 1983; Parker, 1985; Pomeroy, Fewtrell, Butler and Gill, 1978; Tizard and Grad, 1961). Various aspects of caring for a severely handicapped child have been defined as stressful, from the physical burden of care to the emotional disturbance created by the child, and from the disruption of family life to the burden on family finances. In the following pages we shall explore these different aspects of caring and assess their relative importance for the families who took part in our study.

We assessed the stress experienced by mothers of mentally handicapped children by using the Malaise Inventory. This is a well-standardised instrument based on the Cornell Medical Index, which has met adequate standards of validity and reliability in a number of studies (see, for example, Rutter, Graham and Yule, 1970; Cooke, Bradshaw, Glendinning, Baldwin, Lawton and Staden, 1982; Tew and Laurence, 1975; Gath, 1978). In the Malaise Inventory the respondent is asked if he or she suffers from any one of 24 different health problems. Rutter, who obtained mean scores for parents of normal children of 3.12 in the Isle of Wight and 4.15 in London, suggested that scores of greater than 5 or 6 can be considered as outside the normal range, and as evidence of stress.

The mean malaise score for respondents in our study was 5.8, which indicates that many were experiencing a degree of stress. However, variations around this mean were very great. First we hypothesised that levels of stress in the carer might vary with the diagnostic category of the child's handicap. Thus children with Down's syndrome, who are usually communicating and mobile, might be expected to be less stressful for their parents than children with cerebral palsy, who are often immobile and multiply impaired, presenting additional physical burdens. However, when the mean malaise scores of the main diagnostic categories were compared, the differences did not reach significance, and such differences as existed were in the opposite direction to that which one might have expected. Thus the mean malaise score of parents of children with Down's syndrome was the same as the mean score of the whole sample, at 5.8, while the mean score for parents of children suffering from cerebral palsy was slightly lower at 5.1.

Secondly it was hypothesised that it might be the nature of the child's impairment which determined the level of stress in the carer. For example, were children who were incontinent or immobile more likely to cause their parents stress? Analysis showed that neither incontinence nor lack of mobility were associated with higher malaise scores in carers. Were children who could not talk, or who could not care for themselves, more stressful? Here again we found no significant associations between higher malaise scores and either lack of communication skills or lack of self-help skills.

However, combining impairments into a composite score produced a significant association between the number of impairments and malaise. The impairment score was calculated on the basis of data collected from teachers and care assistants in the first stage of the study, using the Disability Assessment Schedule, and was therefore quite independent of the 'stress' variable. The dimensions which were used were those which assessed each child's mobility, continence, self-help skills, sensory impairments, speech, behaviour, quality of social interaction, tendency to have epileptic fits, physical disorders and psychiatric disorders. The impairment score was a rather crude measure, combining as it did both physical and mental impairments and some of their handicapping consequences. However, it did give a rough measure of the multiplicity of a child's impairments, in addition to mental retardation. Each child scored one point for each dimension in which she or he was assessed as being severely impaired. The actual maximum score was 10. Mothers whose children scored 0 or 1 on the impairment scale had a mean malaise score of 5.04; those whose children scored between 2 and 6 had a mean malaise score of 6.03; finally, those whose children were so impaired that they scored 7 and above had a score of 7.00. So multiple impairments in children were associated with significantly more stress in carers.

Thirdly we investigated the relationship between stress and the burden of work involved in the care of the children. For this purpose we created an extra work scale, based on a series of questions which asked whether the child's impairments caused extra work for his or her chief carer. The questions covered cleaning and tidying, cooking, washing clothes, shopping, and other tasks. No extra work was scored as 0, a little extra work as 1, and a lot of extra work as 2, to give a maximum possible score of 10. The results of this analysis are presented in Table 3.3. As this shows, mothers who had a greater burden of extra work because of their handicapped child had very significantly higher malaise scores. These findings are similar to those of Cooke *et al.* (1982). In those families where husbands regularly helped with the care of the child, wives tended to have lower stress scores, especially when the help took the form of taking the child out so that mothers could have a break from caring (Quine and Pahl, 1987).

Table 3.3: Extra work score by malaise scores

Extra work score	Mean malaise scores	Standard deviation	N
0–1	4.59	3.69	59
2–3	5.01	3.87	63
4–10	7.43	4.18	76

p < 0.001; highly significant

Fourthly we investigated the effects on mothers of looking after children with behaviour problems. This term contains within it a variety of characteristics including temper tantrums, destructiveness, night-time disturbance, spitting, biting, screaming, wandering, and sexual delinquency. We have seen that physical impairments, such as immobility or incontinence, were not necessarily related to high malaise scores. However, when we considered behaviour disorders the picture was dramatic. There was a very significant association between the degree to which a child's behaviour was disordered and the level of stress in the carer, as Table 3.4 shows. The more severe the behaviour problems in the child, the more stressed the mother in the carer, as Table 3.4 shows. The more severe the behaviour problems in the child, the more stressed the mother was likely to be: the 82 mothers with children with severe behaviour disorders had a mean malaise score of 7.03, indicating a high level of stress. It is important to remember that the assessment of the child's behaviour was made by the teacher or care assistant in the course of the population study, while the malaise score was calculated on the basis of material collected in the course of the interview with the child's mother. The two measures are thus completely independent of each other.

Table 3.4: Behaviour problems by malaise scores

	Mean malaise scores	Standard deviation	N
No problems	4.66	3.32	78
Mild behaviour problems	5.62	4.40	40
Severe behaviour problems	7.03	4.34	82

$p < 0.001$; highly significant

The link between behaviour disorder and stress is an important finding. However, behaviour disorder is a broad category and we wanted to find out exactly which aspects of the child's behaviour contributed most to stress in the person doing the work of caring. Each carer was asked about a number of different aspects of the management of the child, and their answers were correlated with measures of stress based on the malaise score. The results showed that, in all the areas of daily life at which we looked, children who were more difficult to manage produced more stress in those who cared for them. The highest stress scores were found in mothers whose children were wakeful at night. Some children screamed for hours at night; some were liable to wander out of the house, or to become destructive if not supervised; others simply needed constant physical care, such as the hourly suction with an electric pump which was essential for one child with a tracheostomy. Mothers whose children prevented them from getting enough sleep had a mean stress score of 8.09.

Finally we investigated the effects on mothers of other aspects of family life, only some of which were related to having a mentally handicapped child. We have already seen that having a handicapped child imposed a financial burden on families, both by making it harder for both parents to earn and by causing extra costs. In addition, some of the families had other difficulties to face: 13 per cent were single-parent families; 17 per cent of mothers and 10 per cent of fathers had themselves suffered from ill-health in the preceding year; 40 per cent of respondents said that their home was not suitable for the family's needs, usually because it was too small; 31 per cent had an income of under £5,000 p.a. and 25 per cent said that money was a constant worry.

In order to assess the cumulative effects of economic and social disadvantage we devised an adversity scale which drew together a number of different aspects of hardship. The adversity score took account of the following elements in the lives of our respondents: being a single parent; either husband, wife or sibling having a long-standing disability, or having been an in-patient during the previous year; housing that was unsuitable for the needs of the family; low income; money worries; having an unhappy marriage; lacking a close friend. The adversity score divided the 200 respondents into a high-adversity group of 40, who had four or more of the characteristics which we had used in defining adversity, from a low-adversity group numbering 160 who had three or less characteristics of adversity. The difference between the malaise scores of these two groups was striking. The high-adversity group had a malaise score of 8.6 in contrast to the score of 5.1 of the low-adversity group.

In this chapter we have discussed many different aspects of the lives of families with mentally handicapped children. We have shown that having a handicapped child can impose considerable financial burdens on families. We have documented the extra work involved in caring for a handicapped child and the demands this makes on other family members, but especially mothers. We have described the social isolation which some families experience. Using the Malaise Inventory we have demonstrated the links between multiple impairment, extra work, behaviour problems and adversity, on the one hand, and stress in mothers on the other hand. But how do all these different factors relate to one another? In a book concerned with disorder in the family, which aspects of caring for a mentally handicapped child should we identify as particularly stressful?

In order to answer these and similar questions we constructed a causal model which included all the variables which we hypothesised might be likely to affect maternal stress. We then used a stepwise regression analysis to sort out which variables were important in their own right as direct effects on stress. The result is shown in Table 3.5. It was produced after feeding 28 different variables into the equation. The variables ranged from the child's age and sex, through household income, family composition and parents' employment status, to a variety of different impairments in the child. Of the 28 variables, 19 proved to have little effect on malaise after allowing for the nine in the model. The results of the regression analysis were extremely robust in that feeding slightly different assortments of variables into the analysis did not materially alter the ranking of the variables which appeared to be most significant.

Table 3.5: What factors are associated with stress in mothers? Regression coefficients predicting stress levels

Variables in order of importance	Beta coefficients*	p
Behaviour problems in child	0.24	0.0002
Night-time disturbance	0.23	0.0003
Social isolation of mother	0.21	0.0009
Adversity in family	0.19	0.002
Multiplicity of child's impairments	0.14	0.003
Difficulty in settling at night	0.12	0.05
Child's ill-health	0.11	0.06
Problems with child's appearance	0.11	0.07
Parents have money worries	0.11	0.11

Note: These nine variables together explain 37 per cent of the variance in malaise scores.
*The beta coefficient is a measure of the direct impact of the independent variable when all the other variables are held constant.

Table 3.5 shows that stress in mothers of severely mentally handicapped children is most strongly related to variables falling into two different areas. The first area focuses on the children, and here the most stressful factors are behaviour problems, night-time disturbance, multiplicity of impairments and the child having an unusual appearance. The second area is concerned with the social and economic circumstances of the family, and here the most stressful factors are social isolation, adversity, and worries over money.

HELPING FAMILIES WITH MENTALLY HANDICAPPED CHILDREN

Research on families with mentally handicapped children suggests that they may need help in a number of different areas. In Table 3.6 we set out the parents' answers to the question 'Here is a list of some of the things some parents want more help with. Do you feel that you would like more help to be available?' The answers give some indication of parents' priorities.

Table 3.6: Parents' felt needs for additional help

	Yes	No	Don't know
Advice/information	77	22	1
Financial help	51	48	1
Baby/child sitting	48	52	0
Short-term care	43	56	1
Equipment or aids	34	65	1
Help with household tasks	19	80	1
Full-time residential care	17	80	3

Another series of questions explored parents' feelings about professionals. The answers showed that parents were likely to perceive professionals as helpful when they had specialist knowledge of the problems involved in bringing up handicapped children, when they gave accurate and appropriate advice and information, and when they treated parents with kindness and respect. Professionals were likely to be seen as unhelpful if they appeared to be withholding information, if they lacked knowledge of possible sources of help, or if they treated parents with condescension or rudeness.

Many studies have stressed that families with handicapped children are likely to need financial help, if they are not to be substantially poorer than families without handicapped children. Even though many are in receipt of social security payments aimed at families with handicapped members, they are still likely to be poorer. One long overdue change was the extension of the Invalid Care Allowance to married women in 1986; this benefit is intended to compensate for loss of earnings, but until that date it was paid only to men and to single women, who made up a small proportion of all carers. The provision of adequate income maintenance to people whose capacity to earn is reduced by their responsibility for a handicapped child has been advocated by many researchers (see, for example, Townsend, 1979; Buckle, 1984; Baldwin, 1985; House of Commons, 1985; Parker, 1985).

Many of the problems which families face can be ameliorated by appropriate practical help. Given the heterogeneous nature of mentally handicapped children as a group, the help which their families need is likely to be equally varied. However, the majority of studies stress the value of giving the family some relief from responsibility for caring for the child, whether this takes the form of short-term care, holiday day-care, fostering schemes, or shared care with another family. In addition, there is likely to be a continuing need, for a minority of mentally handicapped children, for longer-term residential care, either in boarding schools or in home-like residential units in the community (Wilkin, 1979; Baldwin and Glendinning, 1983; Parker, 1985). It is very difficult to assess the effectiveness of services in meeting the needs of families. So many variables are involved that it is impossible to be absolutely confident about the effect of any one variable. For example, there were no differences in stress levels between those who did and those who did not use short-term care. However, if we selected only those children who had behaviour disorders, the results suggested that giving short-term care to these children does relieve stress: in families which did not use short-term care mothers had a mean malaise score of 8.00, compared with 6.22 for mothers who used short-term care. The same pattern occurred for children with multiple impairments. This finding has important implications for service providers. It implies that parents with behaviourally disordered or multiply impaired children should have priority in access to short-term care, and that it should be made as easy as possible for these parents to apply for and make use of this sort of care.

Elsewhere in this book it is suggested that self-help and mutual aid may play a valuable role in helping families with problems. What part does self-help play for families with severely mentally handicapped children? Since the 1970s self-help groups have been set up in many different parts of Britain. Some have grown out of voluntary organisations working for better services for mentally handicapped people, while others, such as Contact-a-family and Kith and Kids, are specifically aimed at enabling parents with handicapped children to meet each other (Ward, 1982). The central theme of these groups is that 'a problem shared is a problem halved', and they work from the assumption that parents are able to give each other help and support in a way that professionals cannot: the essence of self-help is mutuality. Some families speak warmly of the part these organisations play in the lives of themselves and their children. However, self-help may not be appropriate for very stressed families coping, for example, with multiply impaired or behaviourally disordered children, often with inadequate financial resources. To suggest that these families should tackle their problems through self-help resembles setting a physically disabled man to pull himself up by his own bootstraps.

Many families welcome forms of help which reflect the idea of partnership between parents and professionals, as recommended by the Warnock Committee (Department of Education and Science, 1978). In some instances professionals have become involved in parents' groups in a leadership or resource role; in other instances parents' workshops have been set up by teachers or other professionals (Cunningham, 1983). Another form of co-operation between parents and professionals is the Portage home teaching scheme. This involves a teacher working with child and parent at home on a weekly basis, following a programme of skill acquisition which is precisely geared to the child's own levels of ability (Pugh, 1981). Portage and other home intervention schemes have now been evaluated and the results suggest that these methods can bring significant gains in achievement and improvements in behaviour for the children involved (Revill and Blunden, 1977; Clements, Bidder, Gardner, Bryant and Grey, 1980).

In recent years important advances have been made in the development of techniques which can help parents both to reduce inappropriate behaviours in the child and also to develop positive new skills (Chazan, 1979: Gath, 1978). Gath reviews some of the literature on the use of parents as therapists for their own children, and concludes that parents can play a valuable role in promoting the development of their mentally handicapped children. An account of home-based treatment from a parent's viewpoint can be found in Fish and Fish (1975). Involving parents in this way may have an indirect effect on stress by giving parents a sense of being able to do something positive for their child, as well as acting on stress in a direct way by reducing the incidence of difficult behaviour. The many different schemes now in existence are reviewed by Ward (1982). Some of these schemes are run by parents for parents; others involve collaboration between parents and professionals. As Mittler has suggested, 'collaboration with parents must in the future be seen as one of the hallmarks of the well trained professional' (Mittler, 1979b, p. 12).

CONCLUSION

At the beginning of this chapter we outlined two models of the family which, explicitly or implicitly, shape much thinking on the topic of families with handicapped members. The research described in this chapter suggests that caring for a mentally handicapped child can be a cause of stress in those who do the work of caring, especially if the child is multiply impaired or behaviourally disordered. However, when one considers the work and the financial costs involved in caring, it is hardly surprising that this should produce some degree of stress even in the most normal of families.

Examining the ways in which families care for severely mentally handicapped children can throw light on the debate about the term 'the family'. This is particularly so at a time when the burden of care is shifting from institutional care to community care, which in effect often means care by the family. As the report of the House of Commons Social Services Committee put it:

> Many witnesses have told the Committee of the sometimes intolerable burden of care that is placed on the families of mentally ill and mentally handicapped people who are living at home. Constant demands may exact a heavy toll on families, and especially on parents. (House of Commons, 1985, p. lxxxvi)

However, the use of the words 'family' and 'parents' disguises the fact that within the family individuals may have very different interests. For severely mentally handicapped children who live at home the family provides most of the care they need. However, this care is not provided without costs, and the costs are not carried equally by all members of the family. There is a real sense in which the needs of family members conflict. For example, the need of the child for constant attention over many years may conflict with the need of the mother to take paid employment and to enjoy a normal social life. As Land said:

> Family members may have quite different and even opposing interests. Resources and responsibilities are not shared equally within the family. Just as the concept of 'the national interest' obscures crucial conflicts of interest within the nation, thus favouring the superordinate in society, the demand to preserve and protect 'the family' is to the advantage of its more powerful and privileged members. (Land, 1978, p. 259)

The evidence presented in this chapter suggests that the burdens of caring for mentally handicapped children are carried overwhelmingly by their mothers, and it is they who pay the price in terms of stress, social isolation and sheer hard work.

REFERENCES

Baldwin, S. (1985) *The costs of caring*, Routledge and Kegan Paul, London

Baldwin, S. and Glendinning, C. (1983) Employment, women and their disabled children. In J. Finch and D. Groves (eds), *A labour of love*, Routledge and Kegan Paul, London

Barrett, M. and McIntosh, M. (1982) *The anti-social family*, Verso Editions, London

Bayley, M.J. (1973) *Mental handicap and community care*, Routledge and Kegan Paul, London

Bradshaw, J. and Lawton, D. (1978) Tracing the causes of stress in families with handicapped children, *British Journal of Social Work 8*, 181-92

Brown, G.W. and Harris, T. (1978) *Social origins of depression*, Tavistock Publications, London

Buckle, J. (1984) *Mental handicap costs more*, Disablement Income Group, London

Burden, R.L. (1980) Measuring the effects of stress on mothers of handicapped infants, *Child: Care, Health and Development, 6*, 111-23

Chazan, M. (1979) Home-based projects. In A.F. Laing (ed.), *Young children with special needs*, University of Swansea, Swansea

Clements, J., Bidder, R.T., Gardner, S., Bryant, G. and Grey, O.P. (1980) A home advisory service for pre-school children with developmental delays, *Child: Care, Health and Development, 6*, 25-33

Close, P. and Collins, R. (1985) *Family and economy in modern society*, Macmillan, London

Cooke, J., Bradshaw, J., Glendinning, C., Baldwin, S., Lawton, D. and Staden, F. (1982) *1970 Cohort: 10 Year Follow-up Study*, Social Policy Research Unit, University of York

Cunningham, C. (1983) Early support and intervention: the HARC infant programme. In P. Mittler and H. McConachie (eds), *Parents, professionals and mentally handicapped people*, Croom Helm, London; Brookline Books, Cambridge, MA

Department of Education and Science (1978) *Special educational needs* (The Warnock Report), Cmnd 7212, HMSO, London

Department of Health and Social Security (1971) *Better services for the mentally handicapped*, Cmnd 4683, HMSO, London

Department of Health and Social Security (1979) *Report of the Committee of Inquiry into Mental Handicap Nursing and Care* (The Jay Report), Cmnd. 7468 I and II, HMSO, London

Fish, R. and Fish, M. (1975) Home based treatment: the parents' report, *Apex, 3*, 4-7

Gath, A. (1978) *Down's syndrome and the family: the early years*, Academic Press, London

Glendinning, C. (1983) *Unshared care: parents and their disabled children*, Routledge and Kegan Paul, London

Hewett, S. with Newson, J. and Newson, E. (1970) *The family and the handicapped child*, George Allen and Unwin, London

Holmes, N., Shah, A. and Wing, L. (1982) The Disability Assessment Schedule: a brief screening device for use with the mentally retarded,

Psychological Medicine, 12, 879-90

House of Commons (1985) *Community care,* Second Report from the Social Services Committee, HC 13-1

Land, H. (1978) Who cares for the family? *Journal of Social Policy, 7,* 3

Martin, J. and Roberts, C. (1984) *Women and employment,* HMSO, London

Mittler, P. (1979a) *People not patients,* Methuen, London

Mittler, P. (1979b) Patterns of partnership between parents and professionals, *Parents' Voice, 29,* 10-12

Pahl, J. and Quine, L. (1984) *Families with mentally handicapped children: a study of stress and of service response,* Health Services Research Unit, University of Kent, Canterbury

Parker, G. (1985) *With due care and attention: a review of research on informal care,* Family Policy Studies Centre, London

Pomeroy, D., Fewtrell, J., Butler, N. and Gill, R. (1978) *Handicapped children: their homes and life-styles,* Department of the Environment, HDD Occasional Paper 4/78

Pugh, G. (1981) *Parents as partners,* National Children's Bureau, London

Quine, L. and Pahl, J. (1987) Examining the causes of stress in families with severely mentally handicapped children, *British Journal of Social Work, 15,* 501-17

Quine, L. and Pahl, J. (1986) Parents with severely mentally handicapped children: marriage and the stress of caring. In R. Chester and P. Divall (eds), *Mental health, illness and handicap in marriage,* National Marriage Guidance Council Research Series, Rugby

Revill, S. and Blunden, R. (1977) *Home training of pre-school children with developmental delay: report of the development and evaluation of the Portage service in South Glamorgan,* Mental Handicap in Wales Applied Research Unit, Cardiff

Rutter, M., Graham, P. and Yule, W. (1970) *A Neuropsychiatric Study in Childhood,* Heinemann, London

Study Commission on the Family (1983) *Families in the future,* Final Report of the Study Commission on the Family, London

Tew, B. and Laurence, K.M. (1975) Some sources of stress found in mothers of spina bifida children, *British Journal of Preventive and Social Medicine, 29,* 27-30

Tew, B., Payne, E.H. and Laurence, K.M. (1974) Must a family with a handicapped child be a handicapped family? *Developmental Medicine and Child Neurology, 16,* Supplement 32, 95-8

Tizard, J. and Grad, J. (1961) *The mentally handicapped and their families,* Oxford University Press, Oxford

Townsend, P. (1979) *Poverty in the United Kingdom,* Penguin Books, Harmondsworth

Ward, L. (1982) *People first: developing services in the community for people with mental handicap,* King's Fund Project Paper number 37, London

Wilkin, D. (1979) *Caring for the mentally handicapped child,* Croom Helm, London

Younghusband, E., Birchall, D., Davie, R. and Kellmer-Pringle, M.K. (1970) *Living with handicap,* The National Bureau for Co-operation in Child Care, London

4

Chronic Physical Disorder in Adults

Keith A. Nichols

Andrew's wife went into unexpected renal failure in 1980, when she was 28 years old. At that time Helen was leading a usual kind of life, devoting herself to caring for their two children who were both under school age, and tending a modest home. This pattern of life instantly became a casualty to her illness. To survive, Helen needed to undergo haemodialysis three times a week and to begin the long training (6 months or more) with her husband to achieve self-sufficiency in the haemodialysis technique in order that home dialysis could become feasible.

In reality this meant a period of 9 months during which Helen would leave home three times a week at 7.30 a.m. to travel to the renal unit and eventually return home at about 6 p.m. During her absence the children were coped with by neighbours, or Andrew's mother. Helen showed all the expected long-term effects of uraemia, being constantly tired, losing much of her muscular power and general mobility (her walking range was about half a mile if interspersed with rests), becoming breathless with any exertion and experiencing episodic disturbances by nausea, headaches and skin irritation. Needless to say, her mood state was variable with periods of much anxiety about the future and depression at her present state. There was a background feeling of anger and resentment at the intrusion of illness into her life. She found dealing with the children a great strain because of her lack of energy, and could only take on light housework. As a final assault on her sense of worth, Helen also found it impossible to continue her sexual relationship with her husband, experiencing the female equivalent of impotency.

For Andrew it was a complex and emotionally fraught time. His burdens were many, since effectively he doubled up as housewife and mother for much of each week as well as learning the skills of venepuncture and the management of haemodialysis. Worse, he had to deal with the experience of watching his partner become dramatically weakened physically, and slowly exhausted psychologically. There were various medical crises which included a failed transplant attempt which caused much grief, and a period of peritoneal dialysis (a completely different method of dialysis based on a bag change method) which was much preferred by Helen but then became unusable because of recurring peritonitis. Equally, the children probably sensed that something was wrong, and that life was full of oddities and mysteries. Mother kept disappearing or was in bed a lot. They were often sent to play elsewhere. Then a machine came and they were not allowed into the room set aside for it, either to visit her when it was running, nor at other times unless one of the parents was present.

Five years elapsed. Helen struggled on. She hated haemodialysis and was shattered when the transplant failed, and again when the short spell of peritoneal dialysis had to be ended. Her will to survive faded, and with this she developed a growing conviction that she was a burden and obstacle, preventing her husband and children living normal, happy lives. If she died sooner rather than later, she once said, their chances of finding a substitute would be much greater. Her death a few months ago was basically self-induced — an end to a lonely, tormented final year.

It is not difficult to see how this family has been damaged by these experiences. Andrew will probably carry emotional scars for a very long while and the development of the children, aged 7 and 9 at Helen's death, will be similarly affected. For 5 years they were a family in disarray, frightened and with many powerful needs for care. Many of those needs went unmet. In addition to these burdens it is my view, from the contact that I had as counsellor with both Andrew and Helen, that further stresses were imposed on them, particularly in the earlier years, from the approach taken by the professional people who cared for them. There was unwitting psychological neglect and the unintended creation of stressing experience by staff who were competent and kindly but not specifically oriented to psychological care.

What is my motive in beginning in this somewhat dramatic style, and in making these assertions? It is simply to remind us that adopting the academic perspective in family studies so often has a powerful effect in distancing people from the actual realities of family suffering, the stark issues, feelings and plain despair which a family like Andrew's must face. Their experiences are recorded in order to keep us mindful of what exists to be dealt with. If our intention is to improve the care offered to the families of seriously ill and injured people, we must return to this without fail.

FAMILIES AND ILLNESS

The task before us, then, is to understand something of the stress and distress which may be brought to a family when one of its members becomes seriously ill or injured. We are searching for some sense of direction and priority for those involved in assisting families to cope with illness, and who need to establish how best to spend the limited resources of the professional services. It is an enormous topic to encompass. The diversity of possible illnesses and injuries, together with the great variability in family structure and situation, make a complete discussion far beyond the scope of one chapter. The issues to be faced, for example, when one of a young couple with three children loses a leg, are enormously different from those, say, of a pair of older people, one of whom is in the late stages of diabetes, and consequently has developed renal failure and retinopathy. Thus, to limit the task to manageable proportions, attention will be directed mainly to the issues concerning the spouse or relative supporting the invalid, rather than the entire family. The impact of childhood illness will not be considered since this is dealt with in Chapter 10. Neither will I consider the elderly, or instances of head injury.

It seems to me something of a pointless task amassing evidence demonstrating that life-threatening or seriously disabling illness and injury can be both frightening and occasionally profoundly disturbing for the partner of the sick person. It is obviously so. We do, though, need to have an awareness of the sources of distress and the time when care is most needed. The case outlined above gave a hint of the high level of involvement in treatment and physical support which the partner of a person surviving by haemodialysis must sustain. It will be useful to extend the information concerning haemodialysis as an example of the kind of stresses that the partner of someone who is seriously ill or injured may be exposed to.

A survey of the psychosocial stressors associated with dialysis was recently undertaken at the Exeter Renal Unit (Nichols and Springford, 1984). This included a section dealing with the supporting relatives, almost all of whom were married partners. These people had all seen a dramatic change in life and were either functioning as dialysis assistants or training to do so. Most were coping, although at some personal cost, particularly in terms of disturbing anxiety (which affected 20 per cent of the sample) during the years after training and the inception of home dialysis.

Most of these people found the first few weeks after the onset of the renal failure to be a time of great fright and confusion. This was mitigated by the regular routine of dialysis and their own involvement with training, which meant regular, lengthy contact with the nursing staff at the training unit 3 days a week. Nevertheless, at the time of inquiry, 23 per cent reported being very tense and worried about the task of venepuncture (placing needles in the dialysand's forearm blood vessels to draw blood into the dialyser) — in fact, in a few instances fear of this task amounted to a phobia. Similarly, 31 per cent were finding that their lives as trainees were made difficult because the teaching was inconsistent and poor in quality, which added stress and frustration and undermined confidence levels which were at times already quite low.

When adequate standards on the part of the dialysand and his or her assistant had been achieved in dialysis techniques, the transition to home dialysis was arranged. For the first few sessions a home sister would be present, her visits and support being tapered off in relation to individual needs. The event of home dialysis was usually much longed for. However, it marked the beginning of a phase of great personal responsibility for the wives, husbands or relatives involved. It was also the beginning of a phase, sometimes many years in length, of being left basically alone to deal with a weakened, rather dependent person, whose dialysis routine trapped the assistant almost to the same extent as the dialysand. These burdens show up in the findings. Thus 46 per cent were worried that they would not cope with likely emergencies during dialysis sessions, 31 per cent felt overly anxious about being in charge of dialysis sessions, worrying that they would do harm or even cause the death of their spouse or relative.

In this particular sample there were no 'casualties' to the training programme. However, Lowry and Atcherson (1980) detailed similar strains and stresses in a parallel study, particularly nervous tension on the part of the spouse, which led to several 'drop-outs' from the training scheme.

Home dialysis meant the loss of regular contact with unit staff. The visits 3 days a week fell to once a month out-patient visits. It was, however, a time when, if anything, *more* support was needed because of the responsibility and general increased pressure on the partner. Readily and quickly available back-up was needed. However, 54 per cent reported themselves reluctant to contact the unit for advice or support 'in case they think we are a nuisance'. There was a sense of being more isolated.

As the full weight of care fell upon the partner, other burdens of a more covert nature developed. Thus, 61 per cent felt depressed at how their spouses had changed, 54 per cent felt exhausted and a good proportion felt trapped, in need of a holiday, resenting the dependency and worried about the effects on the children and friends. A quarter believed their own health to be deteriorating. It was instructive to discover that, of those partners in their training period, 23 per cent felt that the staff did not realise how difficult their lives were. This figure rose to 40 per cent of those well-established on home dialysis when the contact was much reduced. The staff appeared to have a need to see them as doing well, whereas many were struggling badly. This effect was noted by Kaplan De Nour and Czaczkes (1974) who were able to establish that medical staff did seriously overestimate the level of well-being in dialysis families. It was certainly not accurate to say that these people were abandoned because the unit still made a basic provision for them. However, in the later years they clearly felt rather left on their own to cope with this major disaster. The case study by Sealy (1984) graphically illustrates this, relating the history of a young couple with too little information and too little guiding support to survive the demands of home dialysis together.

> Again, though, outward appearances did not represent the real Kevin and on a grey, autumn day he ended his life.
>
> All of us who had cared for him were stunned. It drew us together and, when talking with the nursing staff then, I found for the first time the isolation and distance was broken. The great tragedy is that this genuine contact between the staff and myself came only after Kevin's death — I needed them at the beginning and all the way through.

The partner may well also be somewhat alone within the family itself. As Maurin and Schenkel (1976) report from a study of dialysis, 'there appears to be minimal overt communication between all family members . . . although great concern was expressed there was minimal regard for the needs of the non-afflicted family member'.

It is relevant to draw special attention to this experience of abandonment and isolation. It is clearly quite common where there is a long-term burden of nursing to be undertaken by the partner, or where there is a transfer of intensive hospital support to care by the spouse at home. Thus, for example, Thompson and Haran (1985) investigated the well-being of people living with an amputee. One hundred and nine 'key helpers' (mainly wives) were interviewed, revealing 40 per cent to be at psychological risk. There was a pattern of strain, emotional deterioration, isolation and life beset with difficulties.

Speedling (1982), in an intensive study of families dealing with coronary heart disease, reported how stress, confusion and isolation on the part of the wives greatly increased with the transition from the coronary care unit to home care. The lack of clear guidelines, the absence of clear roles and authority for managing the sick men and, above all, the lack of availability of staff for questioning and seeking supportive guidance undermined them greatly. As those of us having contact with any long-term medical problem will know, the long-term support and guidance of the spouse and closely involved family is a major weak spot. To be left alone to cope with stroke victims, progressive neurological diseases, people who have lost their tongue or larynx from cancer, or whatever form of loss has been suffered, can be a high-stress, long-term event. It is no surprise that Tyler Harper, Davies and Newcome (1983), investigating the circumstances of 92 Welsh families, each caring for a person with Huntington's chorea, found that 82 per cent of the principal family carers reported being distressed, 39.5 per cent were depressed and 21 per cent were taking sedatives.

Stepping back from this detail for a moment, it can be seen that certain principles emerge. First, there is an obvious bi-phasic pattern to the experience of families dealing with seriously ill or injured people. The initial phase has to do with the impact of illness, the fright, the confusion, glimpsing the long-term threats and potential losses, and dealing with the immediate logistics of the care that is required. Later, once the medical crisis is over, or at least the disease is identified and its likely course specified, there comes the second phase in which the family, or more usually the spouse, shoulders the burdens and becomes the care-giver. Now, if things go badly, rather than threat and confusion, the key issues are more often isolation and deprivation, followed by emotional and sometimes physical exhaustion. In this later phase the medical and nursing staff may regard the case as one in which rehabilitation has been achieved: 'the patient is doing well at home'. In relation to this our second principle, therefore, must be that this comfortable, 'case closed', feeling is often a dangerous myth. Where long-term illness, disability or disfigurement is involved, a more accurate perception would be, *'patient at home, partner now at risk'*.

In search of a framework — differences between families

Concerning the initial phase of illness or injury, in the first few days, it is reasonable to make the generalisations given above about the state and needs of the relatives involved. Most do respond to the emergency admission of a spouse, parent or child with some anxiety. Thus a generalised anxiety-diminishing procedure may be used in a broad sweep style. For example, in a recent clinical trial, Bunn and Clarke (1979) demonstrated that brief crisis intervention counselling (in the form of one interview which allowed expression of fears, questioning and provided essential information) with the relatives of seriously ill or injured people 'can reduce their very high levels of diffuse and generalised anxiety'.

The care, during a stay in hospital, of both the sick person and any relative closely involved during a stay in hospital is now better understood. This has been expounded at length elsewhere within a framework which I have called 'psychological care' (Nichols, 1984). However, when we turn our attention to the *long-term* emotional and behavioural consequences of illness for family members, the ground is less well trodden and, to some extent, the generalisations desert us. The problem is that few issues in psychology are straightforward, and the psychology of family functioning in particular is extremely complex, with a whole spectrum of variables to be encompassed. Orford and O'Reilly (1981) illustrate this in clear terms, pointing out that a stressing event such as illness occurs within the context of a unique microculture, the family system. The nature of each family system will, in part, determine how a particular family reacts to illness. For example, the roles of 'dependant' and 'care-giver' may be well developed in a family and should the person taking the dependent role become ill, the resultant 'sick role' will be congruent with the pre-existing pattern of transactions. In fact, on occasions it may prove almost welcome.

Should, however, illness strike in the opposite direction, the person secure in the dependent role will be plunged into precipitate independence and responsibility. Disarray may result, at least until a substitute care-giver is established.

In our search for a framework within which to develop an approach to care, radical differences in family structure and process are therefore an obvious reality to be dealt with. It would not be at all surprising to discover wholly different patterns of functioning in the families of, say, two consecutive admissions to a coronary care unit. Here, though, lies a problem. In recognising the importance of differences between family systems, we also have to deal with the fact that there is not, as yet, a well-validated and generally accepted taxonomy of family systems to assist us in working with these concepts. Some attempts have been made to this end, however. For example, Bowlby-West (1983) writes of twelve common patterns of homeostatic adjustment in families following a death from illness. These include the pattern of 'idealisation', in which the lost figure becomes idealised beyond reality, thus distorting current relationships, and 'infantilisation', in which after a child death a surviving child is over-protected and treated in an inappropriately infantile manner in an attempt to guarantee no more deaths. These are useful clinical impressions but sadly lack empirical support and are recognised by Bowlby-West as not exhaustive of the possibilities. Neither, as an alternative, are there well-established descriptive dimensions by means of which workers in this field *consistently* identify the characteristics of individual families. There has, of course, been progress in developing these. Orford (1980) writes of attempts to unravel the consequences of various family characteristics in alcohol problems, child abuse and psychiatric disorder. In so doing he gives an overview of conceptual development in this field and notes that the descriptive dimensions warm–hostile and control–autonomy recur across various studies. At the same time he questions the adequacy of these dimensions alone, and argues for the inclusion of a factor termed family cohesion which, he believes, is a dimension of major significance. The point here is that high cohesion in a family appears to generate greater stress-resistance and coping ability, probably because it involves stronger mutual support and better collective problem-solving skills.

There is no doubt of the relevance of the family system for those undertaking a professional care-role with families who are struggling with the impact of illness or injury. However, in this early era of research and theoretical development, it has to be said that, while the phenomenon of the family system is known, it is not yet possible to pass on a standard descriptive system which has achieved general acceptance and utilisation. At present researchers use what they as individuals notice and find convenient to work with. We are left noting that the family system must be taken into account but with little that is concrete beyond that. In other words, the value of this material is as a useful reminder of the wide variation between families in their reaction to illness and a spur to flexible thinking with individual families.

In search of a framework — the influence of the individual

As members of a family cope with the physical impact of illness or injury in a close relative, they must also deal with the response which the sick person makes to the event. This may range from depressive withdrawal and collapse, through calm adjustment, to an angry confrontational resistance. In this sense the emotional and perceptual characteristics of the sick person *set tasks* for the family to master. If that person's general perception is of threat and loss, and the perceived personal significance of the illness is taken as highly negative, then these tasks may well prove exceptionally demanding.

This is well illustrated by an example involving a 44-year-old business man. He was distinctive as a personality in terms of his drive and ambition which had led to considerable success. However, he suffered a mild stroke which impaired his speech, slowed him down physically and made him very prone to fatigue. His wife and two daughters expected that, after the initial shock, he would turn his habit of striving for achievements to the task of mastering his handicap and making rapid progress in rehabilitation. This was not so. He became morose, depressed and listless. Social and business contacts were cast off and he made life difficult for the family on a day-to-day basis because of his irritability and refusal to do things for himself. He participated in three therapy sessions, then refused further help. He continued to decline, both physically and psychologically, virtually driving the family into hoping for his death. This did happen, with a second stroke a year later. The family were, of course, stunned and confused. Their lives had earlier been centred on this man's power and energy, and they were horrified and at times guilty about the change in him.

The key to understanding what happened came from the few therapy sessions in which he disclosed how he saw the stroke as being, effectively, his death as a significant person. This was because his sense of worth was closely linked with the trait of competitive striving and the long history of achievement. After the stroke he saw himself as no longer able to compete and achieve in this lifelong pattern. Thus his self-worth collapsed. As is likely with such experiences, he declined under this massive destruction of the all-important self-image. He gave up; a critical psychological state which Schmale (1972) described as the foundation of psychosomatic change leading to physical decline. Here you can see the critical part which this man's reaction to his own illness played in determining what his wife and family had to deal with. In this example the reaction to illness proved more of a hurdle than the stroke itself.

The issue of how attitude to illness influences the behaviour of people during time of illness has received growing amounts of attention, from both an individual and a family perspective. King (1983) has reviewed the field of health beliefs, describing the influence that these have on the general stance towards illness, information-seeking, compliance to treatment and efforts towards rehabilitation. Poll and Kaplan De Nour (1980), for example, investigated the so-called 'locus of control' in people surviving by dialysis. This phrase refers to the extent to which a person feels responsible for, and has some control over, his illness, symptoms and recovery. At the two extremes of this continuum are, respectively, the attribution of considerable personal control (internal locus) and the attribution that there is nothing one could have done to avert illness or can now do to challenge it (external locus of control). Those subjects in Poll and Kaplan De Nour's study who belonged to the internal locus of control group generally fared better, with higher levels of dietary and treatment compliance and greater well-being. Similarly, Greer, Morris and Pettingale (1979) investigated women suffering breast cancer and found that those with a stance which they termed 'fighting spirit' had higher survival rates than those showing 'stoical acceptance' or 'giving up'. By inference, the people in these two studies with the more positive response to their condition will have imposed less burden and emotional strain on their partners.

In search of a framework — illness as a set of tasks

A useful, general framework for bringing some order to the confusion of long-term illness and the myriad patterns of individual response and family reaction is that which construes illness as posing a set of tasks or hurdles to be dealt with. Such an approach has been presented by Moos and Tsu (1977) and Moos (1982). Drawing on the classical 'crisis theory' of Caplan (1964), these authors present an analysis of the demands of serious illness and injury in terms of a set of adaptive tasks, without mastery of which a victim of illness will suffer adverse psychological consequences. Moos's material is largely oriented to the sick person. However, as he points out, the basic ideas are equally applicable to close family members. Accordingly I will summarise the scheme by means of an adapted version emphasising the 'tasks' which challenge the close partner of a sick person. This will, for simplicity, be oriented around the situation affecting the wife of

71

a long-term invalid.

Dealing with the sick person's pain, incapacity or disfigurement

The daily confrontation of pain, or recurrent symptoms such as nausea and muscular weakness, poses a conflict for a partner. To remain supportive she needs to be close and empathic, making contact with and showing recognition of the suffering and experience of her husband. Yet to remain stable and *effective* as a care-giver, she must not become overly identified to the extent that emotional engulfment results, whereupon she will become disturbed by an anxious hypervigilance or collapse into disabling distress. Being so closely involved in the suffering and diminution of a life-partner and, at the same time, able to offer little personally to counter pain, disability and disfigurement is a tense and desperate experience. Survival and adaptation will depend on how a wife manages to resolve the situation. There will have to be some distancing at times and acceptance of the limits to her (or anyone else's) power to bring about change. The initially emotionally traumatic changes, say intractable severe pain after a back injury, have to be accepted as part of daily experience. If she cannot master this required change, she, too, will be disabled and her life stopped in its tracks by an excessive identification with the suffering.

Dealing with the sick person's emotional response

The psychological pain of the seriously ill can have a similarly pervasive and powerful effect. Unless a wife can achieve the subtle combination of empathy, yet with sufficient distance to allow her to separate herself from the feelings, she will lose control of her own emotions and behaviour. I recently met a 63-year-old woman whose husband was bedridden as a result of cerebral vascular insufficiency. He was his 'normal self' but could barely hobble a few yards and sustained several incidents similar to minor strokes each week. She was in a state of great agitation and fatigue and, as an example of her disturbed behaviour, would rush through shopping and run back. The problem was that she had become terrified her husband would need her, and would become frightened and panic while she was out, since this had actually happened on one occasion. Since then she had become so identified with his apprehension at being left alone that she had lost control of her own behaviour and was phobic of being further than calling distance from his bedroom. The task is, therefore, to do with being sufficiently in contact with the distress of another that one understands and can offer genuine support, yet not becoming identified beyond a particular point such that one's own emotional functioning is seriously affected.

Dealing with the hospital environment and treatment procedures

Certain treatments do ask much of a wife supporting a husband. Haemodialysis is perhaps one of the most demanding treatments for the partner since she will be asked to learn the skills of venepuncture, sterile technique, preparation, management and closing down of a haemodialysis machine together with anti-clotting and anti-hypotension procedures. What this means in real terms is that at a time of severe crisis she will have to undertake a course of training in an advanced medical technique. In addition, she must learn to complement the way of life necessary for the dialysand if he is to live for long, including the dietary and drug regime, together with physical and social restrictions. There will be much time spent at the training unit and very many interactions with medical and nursing staff. In other words, success in this task requires the development of a rapport with hospital staff, achieving orientation in the medical environment, learning relevant medical terminology and technique, together with acquiring familiarity with quite complex medical technology. No mean feat.

Naturally the demands differ with different diseases. There may be contact with intensive care, coronary care, a trauma unit, a radiotherapy and chemotherapy unit or a neurological ward, followed perhaps by many months of physiotherapy and out-patient contact. To be comfortable in any of these settings a wife will need to gain sufficient familiarity with the geography of the place, the purpose of the equipment and the different roles that the staff fulfil. She will also need sufficient social ability and assertion to engage the staff in conversation so that she does not leave the unit in ignorance, enraged, confused, frightened or humiliated.

The relatives of seriously ill people often have very clear needs in the situation. Hampe (1975) interviewed the spouses of 27 people who were dying of cancer with a view to identifying their most strongly felt needs. Breu and Dracup (1978) extended this work to wives with husbands seriously ill in a coronary care unit. The partner's major needs were:

to be with the dying/sick person
to be helpful to the dying/sick person
to be assured of the comfort of the dying/sick person
to be informed of the pyshical condition, medical plan and expected course of events

to be informed of the impending death
the need to discharge emotion with other people
the need for comfort and support by family/friends
the need for acceptance, support and comfort by health care
  professionals

In order to meet such needs a partner must develop an awareness of them, and a degree of assertion and negotiating power. Otherwise he or she may be neglected and, while probably being given considerable care, the needs that are truly important will go unmet. Equally, if she is too preoccupied with not 'being a nuisance' to busy staff, she may turn down the opportunity to engage in activities to meet her needs.

It is noticeable (and natural) that the client and relatives involved with a renal unit may initially be uncomfortable, suppressing needs and, although surrounded by caring people, somehow managing not to get truly cared for. After a year or so, however, many have mastered the task. They know who and how to ask, they know how to negotiate and they know how to be angry and assertive when necessary. Such mastery of the environment gives them considerable advantages.

Preserving a positive image of, and positive relationship with, the sick person

In the survey, already mentioned, of stressors affecting the partners of people on dialysis (Nichols and Springford, 1984), many partners agreed that they were 'depressed at how he/she has changed', and that they 'resented the way he/she will not do things for him/herself'. People sometimes change dramatically with illness, perhaps becoming inward-looking, demanding, complaining, regressive, apparently losing the ability to reciprocate caring concern and, overall, being very difficult to get on with. Their partners often become confused and resentful about these changes and lose respect for their spouses as a result. For them, this is a further blow because loss of respect undermines and devalues their long-term effort of care. Without a positive relationship the losses seem more difficult to bear, and the effort has less point. In the survey population this problem sometimes arose because the partners had unrealistic expectations and had not been briefed on the *predictable* changes in personal functioning which affect a proportion of people who are immobilised or disabled. Of course, if a partnership does adapt and there is mutual adjustment to the illness situation, then an opposite effect, best described as positive enhancement of regard and quality of relationship, can occur. This task involves, then, an effort to understand changes in the sick person and to accept new limits to their functioning such that respect is maintained. Equally importantly, the partner must avoid encouraging behaviour which she will eventually resent: this point will be considered in more detail below.

Maintaining other relationships; meeting one's own needs

The wife of a man who is seriously ill easily becomes subject to the same constraints as those which beset her husband. She may feel that, in order to give support and companionship, she too must be bound by the same social and physical handicaps that afflict him. Normally a woman does not need to become withdrawn in the sense that it is a *requirement* of home nursing care. However, preserving personal identity by making sure that her own occupational, social and recreational needs are met rather than suppressed may feel to her like some form of betrayal. Hence the tendency may be towards living the life of a co-invalid. What is required in the successful mastering of this task is a positive effort towards maintaining social contact, physical mobility and continued involvement with the world *despite* her husband's illness. As you may imagine, this requires considerable psychological strength. Expressing support by the voluntary adoption of equivalent social and behavioural handicaps to those of one's ill spouse is a motive which is readily understood, but nevertheless one which can cause great damage to well-being.

One of the most frequently encountered traps for the partners of the chronically ill is that of becoming locked into the 'excessive care' behaviour patterns, and then discovering the hardships, personal losses and entrapment that this can bring. A further aspect which adds to the problem is that social withdrawal probably produces deprivation from informal support. Finlayson (1976) reported that the general well-being of family members dealing with illness (in this instance, heart failure) was related to the extent to which the individuals belonged to and used a supportive network beyond that of the immediate family.

Maintaining a balanced perspective

The practical realities and consequences of illness may harbour considerable threat to the spouse and other family members. How does the employer rect, and what is to happen to income and future income? What response does the local community make, and are the neighbours frightened and inclined to keep their distance, or are they supportive and helpful? Is there a period of loneliness and grief to be faced soon? Anxiety and worry are normal, appropriate reactions to such looming threats but, Moos (1982) argues, the task posed is to assess the threat accurately and to balance this by an equally accurate assessment of personal, family and community resources for help and future development. This means that a heavy investment in denial or, alternatively, an unrealistically threat-laden view of the situation must be seen as failure in mastering the task.

This material is, of course, very much idealistic. It is useful, though, in illustrating why caring for the seriously ill should be seen as a major psycho-social task for close family members. Clearly, a high proportion of people do not achieve mastery in these tasks. Equally clearly, the professional services involved during the time of contact with the hospital, and thereafter, often fall very short in assisting people towards mastery. In fact, one of the most saddening personal discoveries for me in working with seriously ill people has been to find that in many instances no planned assistance is given to relatives at all. It was in no way surprising to read the findings by Hawker (1983) on the manner in which nurses dealt with relatives visiting a hospital ward. Essentially the nurses would employ subtle devices and strategies to *avoid* relatives during visiting time — they certainly did not seek them out with a view to offering assistance.

ASSISTING THE FAMILY — ADVOCACY AND SELF-ADVOCACY

We must now face up to the issue of what exactly helping professionals can do to assist families who are caring for a sick person. Shapiro (1983) asks a similar question following her review concerning families dealing with childhood illness. Her answers are, though, disappointingly non-specific: she writes, for example, of developing family-focused ways of viewing illness, and leading physicians and health care workers to be more sensitive to the needs of the family. Not that these are to be rejected as valid targets, but experience suggests that general exhortation changes little, whereas the introduction of specific new practices which can be encompassed by existing resources may well create movement.

The close family member supporting a sick person needs assistance. When should this begin and what form should it take? Although the typical history is a two-stage event with the sometimes less demanding phase of hospital care being followed by a transition to long-term home care and the subsequent increase of responsibilities and burdens for the supporting family member, we have to recognise that the psychological 'work' for the relative begins with admission, or even before. Thus, the initiation of professional help must begin at the time of the admission to hospital; that is, *nursing, therapist and possibly medical staff must take on responsibility for the well-being of the partner or supporting relative and later, with the transition to home care, ensure that the care is properly transferred to community services or continued by the relevant departments of the hospital.*

Why push further burdens onto hospital staff? There are two good reasons. First, bearing in mind the present structure of the hospital services, it is clear that, since much of the care to be given to close relatives will be in the form of information and education specific to the individual case, then the hospital staff *alone* are in a position to carry out this function. Secondly, if the hospital staff simply conscript family members as ill-prepared, poorly informed, unsupported medical auxiliaries and abandon them in such a position, then they are fostering a form of calculated psychological neglect which inevitably risks secondary illness in the form of psychological disorder, alcohol or drug problems, stress effects and psychosomatic illnesses.

In specifying the nature of the assistance to be given, account has to be taken of the following:

1. Caring for the seriously ill or injured over a period of months or years often turns out to be a high-stress situation. There are many potential stressors including lack of knowledge and information, entrapment, isolation, lack of support, burdensome responsibilities, personal deprivations and emotional strain. Thus, *a stress-reducing approach* is fundamentally important.
2. The spouse or close relative is often expected to play a central long-term role in the psychological and physical care of the sick person, and consequently he or she *must* receive an adequate preparation for the task. This needs to cover:
    (a) the necessary physical care to be given and adequate knowledge of the illness to allow freedom from needless worry and unnecessary dependency on the hospital or GP as a result of unnecessary ignorance;

(b) the possible effects of the illness on the sick person, with special reference to long-term changes in his or her behaviour, attitudes and emotional functioning;

(c) the possible effects of the situation on the *care-giver*, together with a forewarning on likely pitfalls and 'situations to avoid';

(d) induction into the principles of self-care, stress management and self-advocacy as a further insulation against stress. With this there should also be a positive 'permission-giving' communication emphasising that the unit and community staff value this effort on the part of the relative as a reciprocal to their own caring endeavours, not the least reason being that, if the caring family member becomes a casualty too, then everybody involved is put under further strain.

If this preparation is omitted then the seeds of confusion, fearful fantasy, stress and ultimate despair have been sown. It can be depended on that some will germinate.

3. The family member caring for a sick person can only reasonably be expected to be efficient and remain free from stress if he or she also has long-term contact with one of the professional staff who 'represents his or her needs' and is responsible for the provision of information, guidance and support — in other words, when there is a reliable system of advocacy.

Two principles thus emerge, both representing a departure from the current sub-culture of technical medicine operated as a hierarchical authoritarian system. First, the primary objective is to give *care*, not just treatment — this care automatically encompassing those in the family who bear the long-term burden of coping with the sick person. Secondly, the supporting family member should be construed as *an associate of the caring team* and thus be given a clear role, clear status, and offered a free traffic of shared information and education. In other words, the conspiratorial style of dealing with relatives is substituted by a positive effort at caring by informing.

These two principles may seem somewhat idealistic, but in practice much can be achieved at ward level by a small investment of time and the creation of a simple system of education and psychological care for the relative involved. This is best illustrated by an example. Let us take the care of a woman whose husband has developed

Guillain-Barré syndrome at age 25 years (an auto-immune reaction involving the major nerve tracts with consequent massive loss of muscular power and motor activity, recurrent episodes of which may persist for several years). Her husband is admitted to a neurological ward in grave physical distress. She accompanies him to admission and thereafter visits regularly.

We must, for the purposes of illustration, now assume that this is a forward-looking ward which has already introduced a policy of primary nursing (that is, each nurse is responsible for overseeing the total care of a small number of clients) and also that the ward staff have skills in basic psychological care. I have described this kind of work elsewhere (Nichols, 1984, 1985).

On admission the first act of care will be the assignment of a particular nurse to primary care responsibilities with this couple. The nurse (I will assume it is a woman in post) will initially work to make the wife as emotionally comfortable in the situation as is possible and to head off anxiety based on misconceptions or disorientation. Perhaps the most important event will be that the nurse arranges to spend a little time with the wife and to communicate to her that part of the nurse's job is to give assistance in the form of arranging education on the nature of the illness, its effects, its treatment, the likely outcome and the long-term effects that it will have on her husband, both physically and psychologically. The nurse will also convey that she is to act as a support figure to the wife and will seek to act as her advocate in the general conduct of the case. She will therefore invite the wife to contact her when she is needing information, is experiencing difficulties or has requests to make. Lastly, the wife will learn that the staff look to her as someone about to join the team who will ultimately take over in the role of care-giver. She thus has a 'duty' to become as informed as she can and, in turn, has a 'right' to as much information as she can cope with. The underlying message in this first contact is clear. The wife is hearing and experiencing that *she is not going to be alone but has a 'special relationship' with a resource person and teacher who aims to prepare and strengthen her.* This is a vital component of the stress-reducing strategy and can be of profound value to close family members facing this situation.

How this nurse organises her contact with the wife will be governed by the pressures of duties, the history of the case, and the availability of teaching resources such as video-tapes, written material and staff from relevant professions. She will devise a programme to suit the circumstances. The key point is that she does not have to take on all the tasks personally but, rather, work in an integrated, work-sharing way with other nurses and other professionals to ensure that this young woman (together with other family members from other cases) receives adequate instruction, is kept informed of events, intentions, problems and revisions to the medical plan. Her job is to assess the young woman's needs and to make sure that they are met by the total resources of the unit at each stage of the care.

As well as ensuring that this programme of education and information exchange is progressing, the nurse will also monitor the psychological state of the woman, assessing whether additional support is necessary or whether referral to the social worker or clinical psychologist is called for. All this may sound unrealistic in view of the other commitments that nurses have. However, it is worth pointing out that in a busy dialysis unit, just exactly this sort of contact goes on as the partners are trained to assist with home dialysis. The key determinant is whether or not the nurses have accepted a formal extension of their role to include this work and, consequently, whether or not there is a properly devised and implemented scheme of organisation to facilitate it.

As treatment of the husband's condition progresses, different aspects of his care need to be dealt with to promote his wife's understanding and involvement. At times the nurse will want the wife to spend some time with the physiotherapists, learning how to help her husband move and how to help him with exercise and strengthening activity. Also, the wife will need to work with the occupational therapist to agree how to encourage and foster self-help skills in her husband and to tackle the issue of him finding a sense of worth through different activities and involvements despite seriously diminished mobility. Lastly, the nurse will want to arrange for some input from the psychologist or social worker. They will deal with the social and psychological side; both how people may react and change in chronic illness and how the care-giver may respond to these changes. They will also teach the basics of self-care, stress management and self-advocacy. Ideally, part of this will be done in a group setting involving other wives or husbands preparing to care for people suffering similar neurological diseases. The supportive function of contact with other people going through the same experience is usually much appreciated.

As an example of the type of communication which can be used to promote understanding and discussion with a woman in a situation such as that described in this example, I have condensed the content of a typical opening to a short teaching session that would be given to her by the psychologist, social worker or one of the therapists on the team. The real point of this example is to show how important it is to share knowledge in a straightforward, honest manner in an attempt to 'head off' difficulties. It gives direction and permission to exercise self-care.

Because you feel horrified and enormously sad for your husband, you will probably experience a great need to do things for him. It will seem hard to make any demands on him and most likely you will want to do everything for him, tolerate his mood changes uncomplainingly, and sacrifice something of yourself and your own life as a gesture. You will probably feel guilty that you are well and mobile and can continue life normally and, because of this guilt, elect to give up many of your activities in order to be with your husband. There is danger in this for you, though.

Should he be an invalid for a very long time, if you become locked into this pattern then two things might happen. First, you may play a hand in turning your husband into a severely dependent person who will have lost the ability to reciprocate care and effort, and who may drift into being a manipulating, demanding person with a very narrow focus of interest and concerned primarily for his own needs. Secondly, you will have narrowed your own life down so that it is very stressed and you feel dreadfully trapped, exploited and a 'beast of burden'. You will greatly resent your husband's behaviour and demands but feel too guilty to demand change. Things will mount up and the strain on you will increase and could bring very great distress.

From the beginning, then, you must be aware of the need for self-care and be aware of the importance of maintaining your own identity, interests and activities. Although your husband is ill and will be an invalid, you must set up your pattern of living so that he strives for a degree of independence from your constant attention. Before discharge you should discuss this together, perhaps with my help, so that you both agree about the general objective. He needs to understand that in de-stressing your own situation by practising self-care and maintaining your own identity you are not being callous but preserving your ability to go on giving care for a long period. You both need to remind one another about the risks of drifting into an excessive invalid or excessive care-giving pattern.

Thus, in overview, the primary nurse maintains a monitoring role with the spouse or relative who is to support the sick person and co-ordinates the provision of educational and support facilities as required. She has a positive *responsibility* to ensure that people in this situation have the degree of self-advocacy which will allow them to use these facilities to the full. It should be said that this approach is not wholly dependent on the primary nursing scheme but it does require that there is a 'key worker' acting as a co-ordinator and representing the needs of each case. Without this, disorganisation and neglect are virtually unavoidable. Overlying this whole endeavour is the notion of advocacy which, as discussed by Walsh (1985), basically means that the advocate represents the interest of clients as if she were representing her own interests. With this atmosphere, the experiences of the family described at the beginning of this chapter and those of Sealy (1984) would have been much less stressful. If there is serious concern to reduce the distress and neglect commonly found in the relatives of the chronically ill, then there seem few alternatives other than a scheme of this type.

Continuing the care

However, only half the story has been told, because sooner or later discharge and the transfer of care to the spouse or close family member must be instigated. As has been seen, the foundations of preparation and education are put down during the hospital-based phase. However, much of the good done will be undermined unless there is

(a) continuity of care and support by community services;
(b) a proper, informed 'hand-over' by hospital staff to community staff; and
(c) continued open access to the ward for information and guidance.

This latter is as important for the community team, including the GP, as for the care-giver. It is a familiar experience for me to talk with GPs and community nurses who feel that they too have been abandoned with demanding cases without back-up or guidance from the hospitals.

Interestingly, Harrisson (1977) picks up this point very strongly. She studied the families of children with Perthes' disease and cystic fibrosis, seeking also the experiences of the medical social workers and health visitors involved in community care. Harrisson's findings

She studied the families of children with Perthes' disease and cystic fibrosis, seeking also the experiences of the medical social workers and health visitors involved in community care. Harrisson's findings support the general claims which I have made concerning family stress caused by long-term, home-based, physical care, and she recommends interventions which are basically similar, aimed at reducing the damaging effects of insufficient information, education and support. Concerning the business of hand-over and liaison with community staff she writes:

> Details of *all* patients with diagnosis, current or expected treatment and probable length of stay (if known) should be dispatched to the community health centres and general practitioners *on the day of admission.*

> Details of the impending discharge of all patients including details of current and proposed home or out-patient treatment should be relayed to health visitors in a similar way to give them an opportunity to visit the patient in hospital and/or his relatives before discharge.

As care becomes home-based the critical issue centres upon whether or not the community team can continue the scheme of support and advocacy begun at the hospital. Their ability to do so will be greatly enhanced if the relative giving care can also consult directly with her original primary nurse and the supporting team of professional staff should genuine difficulties arise which require specific information of the type which the community team may not have to hand. Apart from this, the main objective for the community team will be to prevent isolation, to repeat the message of self-care and stress management, and offer emotional care and support at a level which opposes a collapse in the family morale and a drift into entrapment and distress.

Speedling (1982) provides a fitting final comment in his conclusions following his intensive study of families involved with a coronary care unit:

> During hospitalisation when patients and families might have been actively seeking answers to questions and strategies for coping with impending changes in their lives, the situation was structured in such a way that they adopted a generally passive orientation. During the first weeks at home, when people were thrust into active roles in the therapeutic process, their lack of preparedness fostered

self-doubt, heightened fear and led to an inappropriate passive dependency on a health care system unprepared to give support during this period.

For my own part I have yet to hear a convincing argument against preventive psychological care and education for the sick person and his or her supporting relative. I have, however, witnessed first-hand the very powerful stress-reducing and problem-avoiding impact which such endeavours can achieve.

REFERENCES

Bowlby-West, L. (1983) The impact of death on the family system, *Journal of Family Therapy*, *5*, 279–94

Breu, C. and Dracup, K. (1978) Helping the spouses of critically ill patients, *American Journal of Nursing*, *78*, 50–3

Bunn, T.A. and Clarke, A.M. (1979) Crisis intervention: an experimental study of the effects of a brief period of counselling on the anxiety of relatives of seriously injured or ill hospital patients, *British Journal of Medical Psychology*, *52*, 191–5

Caplan, G. (1964) *Principles of preventative psychiatry*, Basic Books, New York

Finlayson, A. (1976) Social networks as coping resources: lay help and consultation patterns used by women in husbands' post-infarction career, *Social Science and Medicine*, *10*, 97–103

Greer, S., Morris, T. and Pettingale, K.W. (1979) Psychological response to breast cancer: effect on outcome, *Lancet*, *1*, 785–7

Hampe, S.O. (1975) Needs of the grieving spouse in a hospital setting, *Nursing Research*, *24*, 113–20

Harrisson, S.P. (1977) *Families in stress*, Royal College of Nursing, London

Hawker, R. (1983) Interaction between nurses and patients' relatives. Unpublished Ph.D thesis, University of Exeter, UK

Kaplan De Nour, A. and Czaczkes, J.W. (1974) Bias in assessment of patients on chronic dialysis, *Journal of Psychosomatic Research*, *18*, 217–21

Kaplan De Nour, A. and Czaczkes, J.W. (1976) The influence of a patient's personality on adjustment to chronic dialysis, *Journal of Nervous and Mental Diseases*, *162*, 323–33

King, J.B. (1983) Health beliefs in consultation. In D.A. Pendleton and J.C.Hasler (eds), *Doctor–patient communication*, Academic Press, New York and London

Lowry, M.R. and Atcherson, E. (1980) Home dialysis dropouts, *Journal of Psychosomatic Research*, *24*, 173–8

Maurin, J. and Schenkel, J. (1976) A study of the family unit's response to dialysis, *Journal of Psychosomatic Research*, *20*, 163–8

Moos, R.H. (1982) Coping with acute health crises. In T. Millon, C. Green and R. Meagher (eds), *Handbook of clinical health psychology*, Plenum,

New York

Moos, R.H. and Tsu, V. (1977) The crisis of physical illness. In R.H. Moos (ed.), *Coping with physical illness*, Plenum, New York

Nichols, K.A. (1984) *Psychological care in physical illness*, Croom Helm, London; Charles Press, Philadelphia

Nichols, K.A. (1985) Psychological care by nurses, paramedical and medical staff: essential developments for the general hospitals, *British Journal of Medical Psychology, 58*, 231–40

Nichols, K.A. and Springford, V. (1984) The psycho-social stressors associated with survival by dialysis, *Behaviour Research and Therapy, 22*, 563–74

Orford, J. (1980) The domestic context. In P. Feldman and J. Orford (eds), *Psychological problems — the social context*, Wiley, New York and Chichester

Orford, J. and O'Reilly, P. (1981) Disorders in the family. In S. Duck and R. Gilmour (eds), *Personal relationships*, vol 3, Academic Press, London

Poll, I.B. and Kaplan De Nour, A.(1980) Locus of control and adjustment to chronic haemodialysis, *Psychological Medicine, 10*, 153–7

Schmale, A.H. (1972) Giving up as a final common pathway to changes in health, *Advances in Psychosomatic Medicine, 8*, 20–40

Sealy, L.A. (1984) Alone with illness. In K.A. Nichols (ed.), *Psychological care in physical illness*, Croom Helm, London; Charles Press, Philadelphia

Shapiro, J. (1983) Family reactions and coping strategies in response to the physically ill or handicapped child, *Social Science and Medicine, 17*, 913–31

Speedling, E.J. (1982) *Heart attack — the family response at home and in the hospital*, Tavistock, New York

Thompson, D.M. and Haran, D. (1985) Living with an amputation — the helper, *Social Science and Medicine, 20*, 319–28

Tyler, A., Harper, P.S. Davies, K. and Newcome, R.G. (1983) Family breakdown and stress in Huntington's chorea *Journal of Biosocial Science, 15*, 127–38

Walsh, P. (1985) Speaking up for the patient, *Nursing Times*, 1 May 1985, pp. 24-6

5

Coping with Problem Drinking in the Family

Barbara S. McCrady and William Hay

Problem drinking is one of the most common of the disorders considered in this volume. In the United States an estimated 70 per cent of adults drink, and approximately 10 per cent have drinking problems. The range of definitions of drinking problems is broad, but we generally will follow the diagnostic scheme used in the Diagnostic and Statistical Manual of Mental Disorders (DSM-III, American Psychiatric Association, 1980). In the DSM-III, alcohol problems are divided into organic mental disorders and substance use disorders. The organic mental disorders related to alcohol use refer to the acute and chronic effects of heavy alcohol consumption, including acute alcohol intoxication, alcohol withdrawal syndrome, and alcohol amnestic syndrome. In this chapter, however, we will deal with the substance use disorders, rather than organic mental disorders. Substance use disorders are categorised as *alcohol abuse* or *alcohol dependence*. Alcohol abuse is defined: (1) if a drinking pattern is 'pathological', as evidenced by requiring alcohol for daily functioning, frequent blackouts because of alcohol (memory loss for events while drinking, without loss of consciousness), alternating between periods of abstinence and heavy drinking, or other changes in drinking pattern indicating difficulties; and (2) if an individual experiences life problems because of drinking, such as family problems, job problems, legal problems, or health problems.

A diagnosis of alcohol dependence is appropriate if the individual meets the above criteria for alcohol abuse, and either shows evidence of tolerance to alcohol, or presence of alcohol withdrawal symptoms when the person stops drinking or decreases consumption.

While the stereotype of the alcoholic has been the skidrow 'bum' who has no job, family or adequate housing, epidemiological studies find that the majority of problem drinkers are socially stable and middle class. This superficial social stability belies the pain and chaos experienced in these families. While excessive drinkers are as likely to marry as anyone else in the population, their divorce rate is seven times that of the general population (Paolino, McCrady and Diamond, 1978). Even when couples stay together their marriages are often conflicted and unhappy. Spouse abuse may occur, and spouses may be so affected by living in a family with an alcohol problem that they experience significant emotional problems such as anxiety, depression or psychophysiological problems (Paolino and McCrady, 1977). Family members experience more physical problems, and use health care resources more often than families wihout a problem drinking family member. In the 1940s and 1950s clinicians working with women married to problem drinking men observed these problems, and suggested that their emotional problems predated the drinking problems and indicated deep-seated personality problems. More recent research (reviewed in Paolino and McCrady, 1977) has made it clear that the distress which these women experience is directly related to the disruption and pain that the drinking introduces into the home, and that their problems will diminish if the excessive drinker is able to successfully deal with the drinking problem.

Children growing up with a problem drinking parent are at higher risk than children from other families for developing alcohol problems. Such children suffer from lower self-esteem and school and behavioural problems. Because alcohol problems have such profound effects on the family it is important to develop models of understanding problem drinking that fully integrate the family into the understanding and treatment of these problems.

THE FAMILY IN THE AETIOLOGY OF DRINKING PROBLEMS

Our primary focus in the chapter will be on understanding the current functioning of the family, rather than focusing on historical information. Before turning to this current perspective we will comment briefly on the role of the family in the development of excessive drinking.

Early theories about the development of drinking problems suggested that problem drinkers came from conflicted or disrupted families. More recent longitudinal data (Vaillant, 1983) suggest that there are no major interactional or psychological features that distinguish the families of origin of excessive drinkers from other families. However, longitudinal and cross-sectional studies both find a strong association between excessive drinking in the parents and excessive drinking in the offspring. Genetic and family research programmes have begun to elucidate the nature of the transmission of drinking problems across generations.

A number of studies have attempted to identify a genetic component in the development of drinking problems. The best-known of these studies (Goodwin, Schulsinger, Hermanen, Guze and Winokur, 1973) examined drinking problems in offspring of excessive drinkers who were adopted away from their natural parents at birth. Using such a sample allowed the investigators to examine the association between drinking problems in the offspring, drinking problems in the biological parents (from whom the children received their genetic inheritance) and drinking problems in the adoptive parents (from whom the children received their strongest models of drinking behaviour). When considering the most serious forms of drinking problems, Goodwin's research group found a strong association between drinking problems in the biological parents and drinking problems in the offspring, and virtually no association between adoptive parents' and children's drinking problems. Later studies (e.g. Bohman, Sigvardsson and Cloninger, 1981) have found similar results, leading to the conclusion that certain kinds of drinking problems have a strong genetic component, while others appear to be more environmentally determined.

One environmental factor that appears to have a significant relationship to the development of drinking problems in the children is the structure and stability of the family. Wolin, Bennett, Noonan and Teitelbaum, have studied family rituals, 'a symbolic form of communication which, owing to the satisfaction that family members experience through its repetition, is acted out in a systematic fashion over time' (Wolin et al., 1980, p. 201). Rituals develop 'as the family attempts to carry out its plans for everyday activities such as meals, as it marks transitions such as birth, graduation, marriage and death, and as it makes arrangements for special events such as holidays' (Wolin et al., 1980, p. 201). To study family rituals, Wolin and Bennett's research group interviewed 25 families with at least one parent who had a drinking problem. They assessed how families behaved around several areas associated with family rituals, such as mealtimes, holidays and vacations, coded the degree to which these events were ritualised, and evaluated the degree to which these rituals were disrupted by the problem drinker.

The relationship between stability of the family's rituals in the face of excessive drinking and drinking problems in the children was quite notable: two-thirds of the families with an adult child with a drinking problem had markedly altered their rituals because of the drinking ('subsumptive' rituals), while only 8 per cent of the families without a problem drinking offspring had 'subsumptive' rituals. The results suggest that a family's ability to maintain the same kinds of structures, order, predictability and connectedness, in the face of a significant drinking problem in one family member, is an important variable in the transmission of drinking problems across generations, even when the children may be genetically at risk for the development of drinking problems.

THE PHENOMENOLOGY OF THE ALCOHOL-TROUBLED FAMILY

Before turning to a formal model for describing the interactions between excessive drinking and the family, it is important to consider the experiences of a family with a member who is drinking heavily and problematically. The most lucid description of this phenomenology was provided by Joan Jackson (1954), following intensive interviews with members of Alanon who were wives of men with drinking problems. Because of the source of her data, they tell us little about the experiences of families with a problem drinking mother, and little about the experiences of families who do not feel the need for outside support and help to cope with their problems. Thus the description that follows is probably most relevant to families where the father is the excessive drinker, and whose drinking pattern is one of daily drinking and loss of control.

When a family member first begins to change his/her drinking pattern the change may be subtle, and not easily discerned. Occasional drunkenness, staying out too late, or doing embarrassing things in public may be ignored, or explained away by considering current life stresses or problems. Family members may express concerns to the drinker, or to friends or family members. These concerns are likely to be brushed away, and the behaviour explained as normal. However, if the person's drinking becomes more frequent, or the problems become more serious, the family become unable to normalise them. The drinker may do things which the family do not understand, and which are upsetting. He or she may be experiencing alcoholic blackouts, and not remember conversations held or promises made. This introduces a sense of uncertainty into the family, leading each family member to wonder if he or she misheard or misunderstood conversations. Even if they are sure that a conversation transpired, they may not understand why the drinker is denying that it occurred. They may think that the drinker is lying or does not care. This experience is particularly difficult for children, who look to their parents for stability and predictability. Chronic heavy alcohol consumption also has major effects on the drinker's mood, and these effects may vary with blood alcohol level. Thus the drinker may oscillate between anger and depression, or anxiety and fatigue. His or her mood is unpredictable, and the family do not know what to expect from day to day. The drinker may be experiencing withdrawal symptoms, and be tremulous, nauseous or have serious sleep difficulties. To the family who know little about alcohol dependence these symptoms may be frightening, and a cause for serious concern about the drinker's health. Thus, as the drinking becomes more frequent and heavy, the family begin to experience a sense of unpredictability about their home — plans are made and broken, tempers flare, behaviour is mercurial and worry blankets the family.

As the family become more aware of the cause of these changes, they begin to try to find ways to help and to cope. Initially they may hope that 'understanding' and decreasing pressure on the drinker may help. Thus families may assume some of the drinker's responsibilities, try to avoid arguments or discussing problems that might be upsetting, and be kind and concerned when the drinker is sick. These behaviours are probably *normative* ways for a healthy family to respond when one member is ill, and these actions are usually helpful and supportive to a sick family member. Unfortunately, in alcohol-troubled families these kinds of reactions may instead exacerbate the drinking problem, by removing aversive consequences of drinking, and may eventuate in more serious family problems as the excessive drinking begins to create new problems (e.g. financial or job problems or physical abuse).

As these efforts to help fail, the family may begin to try to control the person's drinking. Searching out bottles of alcohol and pouring them down the drain, going down to the local pub to bring the father home, taking the drinker's name off the cheque book, locking the liquor cabinet and hiding the car keys are all attempts to control the person's access to alcohol. In some families these efforts may be successful, and prevent drinking. As often, however, such actions anger and frustrate the problem drinker, who finds other ways to obtain alcohol, and may drink to retaliate against these attempts at control.

Over time, families may diverge in the course which they take. Some may decide that they cannot continue to function with the excessive drinker as part of the family, and the spouse may effect a separation or divorce. Others may decide that maintaining the family as a unit is crucial to them (for religious or personal value reasons), and try to find a way to cope with the chronic problems which they experience. They may accept that they cannot control or change the excessive drinker's behaviour, and develop a pattern of family life that minimally involves the drinker and is minimally disrupted by his/her drinking. The family may decide that their own efforts at control have been ineffective, and want to put an all-out effort into getting the drinker to seek treatment. The spouse may set an ultimatum ('get treatment or I will leave'); the family may set up an intensive confrontation with the drinker (Johnson, 1973), or the family may change their patterns of reacting to the drinking, by discontinuing controlling behaviours, allowing the drinker to experience the variety of naturally occurring aversive consequences of drinking, and by providing clear feedback about the effects the drinking is having on them.

Through these efforts, or because of other external pressures, the excessive drinker may decide to stop drinking. With or without treatment, long-term success rates are poor for continuous abstinence or continuous moderated use of alcohol. Thus even the decision to seek treatment is more likely to meet with repeated difficulties than with immediate success. Part of the reason for the difficulties with long-term maintenance of change may be due to the physiological changes that occur after chronic heavy alcohol consumption, but many of the difficulties come from the variety of life problems which the drinker encounters. Family problems tend to accumulate when one family member is drinking heavily. Debts accrue, sexual problems develop, behavioural and school problems of the children go untended, and hurt and angry feelings accumulate between the partners. The family may never have developed, or may have lost, their ability to communicate effectively. Thus the newly sober excessive drinker is confronted with a range of family problems, and is ill-equipped to deal with them effectively. Not surprisingly, many relapses occur in response to family or other interpersonal stresses, as the drinker returns to familiar ways of responding to difficult situations.

Sharon and Don illustrate many of the problems described in this section. Sharon, a 41-year-old school teacher, and Don, a 46-year-old small businessman, had many years of difficulties before seeking treatment for Sharon's excessive drinking. Sharon had been a daily drinker for 7 years prior to seeking treatment, but her family had been aware of this problem for only a year. She drank heavily before and after school, and usually was home in bed when Don and their three children came home from work and after-school activities. At times she was asleep; and other times she was groggy, her speech was slurred, and she seemed somewhat incoherent. Don was convinced that Sharon had a serious medical problem, and took her to a succession of physicians for evaluation. Each came up with negative findings, but Don continued to fear that his wife was dying from a brain tumour or other neurological disorder. Sharon's youngest daughter, Melanie, knew that her mother was drinking, but was sworn to secrecy.

Finally, Don began to realise that he smelled alcohol on Sharon's breath, and began to confront her about her drinking. She vehemently denied drinking, even though she was functioning poorly, missing work, not caring for the house and drinking more heavily. As Don became aware of her drinking, he and the two older boys, Marc and Stephen, became obsessed with trying to get her to stop drinking. Don would organise 'bottle hunts' in the evening, and he and the boys would spread out through the house, seeking out hidden liquor bottles. Don, who had a quick temper, began to get into physical fights with Sharon, which often began when he would help her get to the bathroom when she was intoxicated. She would stumble or stagger, and he would be rough with her, often provoking her to shove him, with his responding with a shove or slap.

At the same time Don was attempting to take more of the responsibility for their children. Marc, the eldest, had mild learning problems, which necessitated frequent visits to his school, and conferences with the teacher. Don took time away from his business for these visits, and became increasingly angry with Marc for being disabled, and with Sharon for not doing something that he saw as her responsibility. He had frequent outbursts at home, which contributed to Sharon's drinking more and more.

The family finally forced Sharon to seek treatment after Melanie found her mother unconsciousness when she came home from school. She immediately called her father, who arranged for an ambulance to transport her to a local hospital with an alcohol treatment programme.

In this section we have described the subjective experience of families with an excessive drinker. As we cautioned at the beginning, this is only one possible phenomenology, and individual families may experience excessive drinking quite differently. However, this description does give the reader a sense of what happens in the families of problem drinkers. We will now turn to our formal model for analysing excessive drinking and the familial context of excessive drinking.

MODEL FOR CONCEPTUALISING EXCESSIVE DRINKING AND THE FAMILY

Although the focus of this book is on the family context of disorders, we believe that excessive drinking is both an individual *and* a family problem, and that a comprehensive model must take both into account. We assume that there are multiple pathways for the development of drinking problems — some related to the family, some independent of the family. Similarly, we assume that recovery from drinking problems requires attention to the individual needs and problems of the excessive drinker, the relationships that the excessive drinker has with other interpersonal systems (such as the work system, or friends), as well as the needs and problems of the family as a unit. Thus, good family treatment for excessive drinking must include a careful assessment of the individual factors associated with the problem drinker's drinking, and treatment interventions that address those individual factors, as well as careful assessment and attention to the family.

A basic behavioural model is used for understanding drinking behaviour. The model assumes that drinking is preceded by identifiable environmental events which increase the likelihood of drinking. These environmental events may be called *antecedent stimuli, cues* or *triggers* for drinking. These environmental events may relate primarily to the individual excessive drinker, such as particular times of the day, days of the week, or geographical settings which the drinker associates with drinking. Antecedents to drinking may also arise from the family, either in how the family is trying to cope with drinking, or from general problems in the family.

The second assumption of the model is that people react to environmental events with thoughts, feelings and physical reactions. These internal reactions, called *organismic responses*, form the immediate antecedent to drinking.

The third assumption of the model is that events that occur after drinking, or *consequences*, may either perpetuate or decrease drinking. The consequences that occur after drinking may be primarily individual, such as feeling more relaxed in a social setting, or quelling alcohol withdrawal symptoms. However, important consequences occur within the family, which help to maintain and perpetuate the cycle of excessive drinking and disrupted family functioning.

In the following sections we will detail ways that family actions serve as antecedents to drinking, and/or provide positive consequences to drinking. We will also consider the ways that the excessive drinker reacts to these family behaviours. We will first consider how the family copes with drinking, then consider in general how families with excessive drinkers function.

THE INTERPERSONAL FAMILY SYSTEM

Family systems may contain a number of members, including the spouse, children, parents, siblings and other more distant relatives. Determining what family members are involved with the problem drinker's drinking requires complex clinical judgements. This section discriminates between alcohol-focused family involvement and more general connections between family functioning and the problem drinker's drinking. While this may seem an artificial distinction to make, we find it useful in clinical case conceptualisation.

Alcohol-specific influences

Any family member may engage in behaviours that are directly related to the problem drinker's drinking. However, the behaviour of the spouse has been the focus of the most research and clinical speculation.

In clinical settings, spouses report a variety of actions that appear to be antecedents to drinking. Some of these behaviours can be described as 'nagging' the drinker about drinking, and others are better described as 'control' behaviours. Both of these occur at a high frequency among wives of problem drinking men (Orford, Guthrie, Nicholls, Oppenheimer, Egert and Hensman, 1975).

Spouses and other family members may drink with the excessive drinker, and alcohol may be an integral part of some family celebrations. While data are scanty about the actual functional relationship between 'nagging' or 'control' behaviours and drinking, it is of note that in a study of problem drinking men seeking treatment, 74 per cent of their wives reported that they had stopped trying to control the drinking behaviour prior to the man seeking treatment (Djukanovic, Milosavcevic and Jovanovic, 1976).

Organismic variables related to the family are unresearched. The excessive drinker might have strong cognitive and emotional responses to nagging and control behaviours. Cognitive responses might include thoughts of retaliation ('just let her try to control me') or decreased self-esteem ('I can't even stay sober without outside intervention'); affective responses might include anger, depression, anxiety or guilt. The problem drinker may have low self-efficacy expectations about his or her ability to cope with these family behaviours without drinking, and may feel obliged to drink at family gatherings or with certain family members.

The effects of family behaviours on drinking can be speculated upon. It is possible that family actions result in an increase in secretive drinking in order to avoid the unpleasant cues, and may, as a corollary, be associated with gulping drinks, and drinking beverages with high alcohol content. Spouse antecedents may also lead to increased time apart for the couple, resulting in the excessive drinker's drinking coming more under the influence of others who are heavy drinkers.

Family actions which occur during or after drinking fall into three categories: reinforcement for drinking through attention or caretaking, shielding the problem drinker from experiencing negative consequences of drinking, and punishing drinking behaviour.

Victoria D. and her family illustrate the interrelationships between drinking and the family's attempts to cope with drinking. Mrs D. was a 72-year-old woman, admitted to a general medical hospital because of a fall in her apartment, and general malnutrition. She lived alone, following the death of her husband 18 months previously. Mrs D.'s son and daughter-in-law, Peter and Lynn, lived nearby, and they all saw each other frequently. Mrs D. was a daily drinker, and her son and his wife were concerned about the effects of her drinking on her health. Peter refused to discuss his mother's drinking as he felt that it brought shame to the family to have a drunken mother. Lynn often told Mrs D. that the drinking was bad for her, and urged her to quit. Mrs D. was quite hurt by these comments, and felt that Lynn didn't love her. This feeling added to her feelings of loneliness, which she ameliorated by drinking more. Lynn also talked to several of Mrs D.'s friends at the Senior Citizens Center. The friends had noticed the odour of alcohol on Mrs D.'s breath, and Lynn encouraged them to say something to her mother as well. When they did, Mrs D. was even more upset, felt humiliated, and stopped going to the Senior Citizens Center. Her increased isolation fed her feelings of depression, which led to further drinking.

In this family Mrs D. had many individual issues which fed her drinking, including her isolation and loneliness after her husband's death. Thus some of the origins of her excessive drinking were not related to her current family. However, the family in a well-meaning and concerned attempt to get her to stop drinking, provided cues for further drinking, both by commenting directly on the drinking, and by precipitating Mrs D.'s leaving the Senior Citizen's Center where she had some social contacts. Thus, family actions, which were intended to help, instead led to further and heavier drinking.

General family influences

Systems theorists have postulated an intimate relationship between family functioning and alcohol abuse. Early writings focused on the postulated 'need' that the problem drinking family had for a dysfunctional member, while more recent work has described the communication patterns and family structures of families when the excessive drinker is sober or drinking (Steinglass, 1981). Before turning to studies that analyse drinking and family functioning from a behavioural perspective, we will consider Steinglass's work.

Steinglass (1979, 1981) has suggested that 'alcohol plays such a central role in the life of these families that it has become an organizing principle for interactional behavior' (Steinglass, 1981, p. 578). He assumes that family interactional behaviour is intimately connected with the presence or absence of alcohol consumption by the excessive drinker. In his research he studied a group of 31 families which contained at least one excessive drinking parent, observing their interactions at home and in a structured laboratory setting.

At home, Steinglass (1981) observed different patterns of interaction, depending on whether the excessive drinker remained abstinent during the 6 months of the study, continued to drink, or transitioned from one drinking status to the other. He found that families differed significantly on two dimensions of family functioning. 'Distance regulation' measured how the family used space in the home, the degree to which they interacted with each other when they were in the same part of the home, how close together or far apart they were when interacting, and how much time they spent alone. 'Dry' families were relatively flexible in distance regulation, sometimes being apart, sometimes together. In contrast, 'transitional' families were high on distance regulation, suggesting that they spent more time together, and closer together. 'Wet' families were low on distance regulation, suggesting that they were apart most of the time, rather than interacting with each other.

The second dimension that discriminated the families, 'content variability', measured the affective level of family interactions and the variability of both affect and content of interactions over time. 'Dry' families were highest on this dimension; 'wet' families were lower, and 'transitional' families were lower still.

The behaviour of these families in the laboratory (Steinglass, 1979) echoed their interactions at home. 'Wet' families acted independently of each other, while 'dry' families functioned as a family unit to solve problems presented to them in the laboratory.

Taken as a whole, Steinglass's research suggests that families differ significantly, depending on the drinking status of the problem drinker. When s/he is actively drinking the family functions poorly as a unit, with each family member concentrating on independent activities, and relying little on the family for decision-making or support. When the drinker is abstinent the family emphasise family unity and co-ordinated decision-making, although the family also allow for some flexibility and independence for individual family members. What is not clear from Steinglass's work is whether family interactions *change* as the drinker goes from a wet to a dry state, or whether the difference he noted among the different families reflected stable patterns of interaction characteristic of the particular families he was studying. We will consider the implications of these findings for the behavioural model after considering some of the other interactional studies. The remainder of the studies to be discussed have focused on the marital unit, rather than the whole family.

Problem drinker couples are postulated to have poor communication and problem-solving skills. They are seen as rarely being positive with each other, and evolving, over the years, a mode of interacting that involves attempts to control each other coercively, through threats or nagging. As the aversive situation has escalated over time, communication is believed to become more ambiguous, vague and inconsistent. As a result of these poor communication skills and ineffective methods of control, a large backlog of problems accumulates.

A fairly large body of empirical literature supports this description of the marital relationships of problem drinkers. Controlled studies of couples' interactions have found a high frequency of hostile and/or coercive verbal interactions, a paucity of effective communication skills, and a generally low rate of verbal output (Billings, Kessler, Gomberg and Weiner, 1979; Cvitkovic, 1979; Klein, 1979). A lack of intimate, positive exchanges and spending little free time together have also been observed (Djukanovic *et al.*, 1976; Foy, Miller and Eisler, 1975). No studies, however, have examined the influence of these aversive marital exchanges on drinking.

Internal reactions, or organismic variables, probably play a major role in the chain of events which occur after an aversive marital exchange. The excessive drinker may think of drinking as a way to retaliate, or may expect that drinking might strengthen his/her ability to argue effectively. The excessive drinker may, conversely, feel hopeless about the possibility of resolving the couple's problems, and believe that drinking would provide an escape from the unpleasantness of the situation. Affective responses might include anger, depression or anxiety, and the excessive drinker might expect relief from these feelings through drinking.

How these family interactions actually affect drinking is unstudied. The aversive interactions may result in increased secretive drinking, more rapid drinking and avoidance of certain family members.

Family responses to drinking are varied, and some strongly reinforce drinking. One or both partners may markedly change their behaviour during drinking, resulting in positive exchanges not present during non-drinking interactions. The exessive drinking member of the couple may increase his/her assertive or aggressive responses, which might reinforce the drinking (Cvitkovic, 1979). Problem-solving behaviour might also increase (Frankenstein, 1982), and, while drinking, problem drinkers might increase the rate and amount of verbal output when talking to their spouses (Billings *et al.*, 1979). It should be noted that some studies have not noted these improvements in the problem drinker's marital communications while drinking.

Steinglass's work suggests, in addition to looking at specific behavioural sequences, that the interrelationships between drinking and overall family structure must be considered. Drinking has aversive consequences for family functioning, leading to a deterioration of the family's ability to function co-operatively and as a family unit. This poor ability to function as a family unit may serve as an antecedent to further drinking, as conflicts are likely, and the family is poorly able to function as a cohesive whole to deal with family problems.

Cary and Beth's relationship illustrates the poor family functioning described in this section. Cary, 42, was a slim, attractive man, who dressed in stylish clothes, and maintained a suntan all year round. He worked as the director of a community mental health centre. Beth, also 42, was painfully thin, had a heavily lined face, hair dyed a slightly orange tinge, and looked considerably older than her actual age. She worked as the director of nursing at a local hospital.

The couple sought treatment at Beth's urging, because of her concerns about Cary's drinking and their deteriorating marriage. When interviewed together it became apparent that the relationship was indeed distressed. As they began to discuss Cary's drinking, he became angry, red in the face, and said, 'Well, I guess we won't say anything about *your* drinking here.' Beth sniped back, 'At least I don't have anyone on the side. Do you think I don't know what you're up to?' They exchanged insults for as long as the therapist allowed them to do so. As they talked, they revealed that they owned a second home, near the local beaches. Cary frequently went to stay at this home for days on end. Beth was certain that he drank and carried on with other women while there. In turn, Cary was clear that he intensely disliked Beth, and spent time at the other home to avoid her. He cited her constant nagging and criticism, what he perceived as her self-righteousness about alcohol (when he thought that she also drank heavily), and her physical unattractiveness as reasons to stay away. Beth said Cary was physically abusive and verbally vicious when drinking, and described her 'nagging' as attempts to get him to stop drinking. She also blamed him for her physical appearance, saying that his problems were so stressful to her that she couldn't eat, and didn't care about the way she looked.

Cary and Beth present an extreme example of the kind of negative and hostile relationship that can develop in marriages where excessive drinking is present. They devoted their interpersonal energies to 'one-upping' the other in cruelty, and each placed all blame for the problems on the other. They were completely unable to discuss a problem collaboratively, and certainly unable to solve any of the serious problems between them. There is no way to know how their relationship was before drinking became a problem, because their perceptions of their entire marriage were negatively clouded by their current anger.

IMPLICATIONS FOR ASSESSMENT AND TREATMENT

The behavioural model has wide-ranging implications for the assessment and treatment of excessive drinking. The model also provides a framework for plotting future research directions, although that is beyond the scope of this chapter.

Assessment implications

A comprehensive assessment requires attention to problems at various levels, including the individual or intrapersonal level, the family level, and the interpersonal level. In addition, the clinician must attend to problems directly related to drinking, and to more general life problems of the individual and the family. Conceptually, Figure 5.1 illustrates the potential areas for comprehensive assessment of a problem drinker and family who present for treatment. Table 5.1 provides examples of the kinds of problems that might be examined at the various levels of assessment and treatment. We will focus our discussion on assessment and treatment at the family level, but urge the clinician not to overlook these other important areas for treatment.

Figure 5.1: Behavioural matrix to describe drinking across multiple life systems

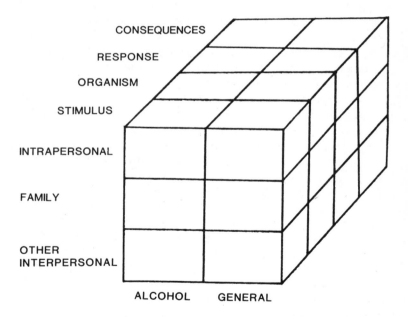

Evaluation should include several types of assessment. Careful interviewing forms the basis of the initial assessment, and should include the excessive drinker and at least one family member. The goals of the initial interview are to establish rapport, gather information about problems that might require immediate attention (such as physical abuse, need for alcohol detoxification, or need for attention to an acute physical problem), and begin to assess the problems associated with drinking and the family's functioning. (See McCrady, 1985, for a more detailed discussion of individual factors to be assessed at the beginning of treatment.)

Structured procedures can be used to collect more systematic information. Self-monitoring cards can be used by the excessive drinker to record daily alcohol intake, subjective urges to drink, situational aspects of drinking and urges, and marital satisfaction. Self-monitoring cards are given to clients to use between treatment sessions. Spouses can also be enlisted in the monitoring process, and can keep daily records of their partner's alcohol consumption, their own actions related to drinking, their marital satisfaction, or other behaviours being targeted during therapy (McCrady, 1982). Clients (we are referring to any family member involved in the treatment as a client) are instructed to carry cards with them at all times, and to make entries on the card whenever the behaviour or feeling being monitored occurs. The use of self-monitoring cards has several advantages: (1) they allow clients to develop a more accurate picture of their own problems; (2) they help clients become more objective about their own problems, by learning how to be self-observant, rather than just engaging in the behaviour; (3) they provide the therapist a more accurate picture of the clients' problems; (4) they help clients and therapist alike to identify specific antecedents and consequences of drinking, facilitating the assessment of the relationship between drinking and family problems.

Behaviourally specific questionnaires such as the Drinking Antecedents and Consequences Questionnaire (DACQ) (Zitter and McCrady, 1979) or the Spouse Behavior Questionnaire (SBQ) (Orford et al., 1975) provide important information about the relationship between drinking and a variety of individual and spouse behaviours. The DACQ lists approximately 260 situations which could be antecedents to drinking. The situations are divided into ten areas: Environmental, Work, Financial, Physiological, Interpersonal, Marital, Parents, Children, Emotional, and Major life stresses. In addition, sections at the end of the questionnaire ask about positive and negative consequences of drinking, as perceived by the excessive drinker. Using the DACQ allows the therapist to do a comprehensive assessment of situational antecedents of drinking, provides the excessive drinker an opportunity to think about his/her drinking rather broadly and provides the therapist with a detailed picture of the relationship between drinking and family problems.

Table 5.1: Behavioural Matrix of Influences on Drinking

	Antecedents	Organismic	Response	Positive consequences
Intrapersonal				
Alcohol-specific	Time Drinking settings Alcohol	Withdrawal symptoms Cravings Positive expectancies for alcohol use Negative affect	Drinking	Decreased withdrawal Decreased negative affect Decreased craving
General	Life stressors Work pressure Failure situations	Negative self- evaluations Low efficacy expectations Positive expectancies for alcohol use Negative affect Craving	Drinking	Decreased negative affect Euphoria Decreased self-awareness Forgetting
Interpersonal — *family*				
Alcohol-specific	Family drinking Family celebrations 'Nagging' Attempts to control drinking	Negative affect Retaliatory thoughts Low efficacy expectations Feeling obligated	Drinking	Family attention when drinking Taking over responsibilities Shielding from negative consequences

	Antecedents	Organismic	Response	Positive consequences
General	Poor communication and problem-solving Coercive control Vague and inconsistent communication Marital problems Child problems Conflict with parents	Retaliatory thoughts Negative affect Expectation of increased assertion Feelings of failure	Drinking	Increased affection Increased assertion Increased verbal output Decreased negative self-awareness Increased problem-solving
Other interpersonal Alcohol-specific	Others drinking Offers of alcohol Social pressure to drink Business/social meetings Parties	Cravings Positive expectancies for alcohol use Embarrassment Social discomfort Low efficacy expectations	Drinking	Decreased craving Increased social comfort Decreased negative self-evaluations
General	Social situations Problems with friends Problems with supervisors Problems with co-workers	Negative affect Negative self-evaluations Expectation of increased assertion Expectation of decreased social anxiety	Drinking	Decreased social anxiety Increased assertion Problem avoidance

The SBQ lists about 60 behaviours that spouses engage in to cope with drinking. The behaviours include many of those described above as either antecedents or consequences of drinking. Using the SBQ allows the spouse, excessive drinker and therapist to assess the degree to which the spouse has been attempting to cope with drinking, and also identifies the types of coping attempted. Clinical interviewing based on the SBQ responses often helps clarify for the spouse the ineffective or counterproductive nature of many of the ways he or she has used to attempt to cope.

Direct observation of the family or couple while interacting provides the therapist with rich information about the current functioning of the family. Observing the family can help the therapist assess how information is communicated in the family, how the family deal with emotional issues, how they solve problems, and what kinds of problems exist in these areas. These observations may be video-taped and coded according to structured coding systems, such as the Marital Interaction Coding System (MICS — Hops, Wills, Patterson and Weiss, 1971), allowing the therapist to have detailed information about a range of communication skills and deficits.

Self-report questionnaires complement the direct observations which the therapist can make in the treatment session. They can be used to assess how happy each partner is with the relationship, what specific problem areas are of concern to each partner and how family members perceive the ways that the family handle various emotional and practical tasks of family living. The Locke–Wallace Marital Adjustment Test (MAT — Locke and Wallace, 1959), the Areas of Change Questionnaire (Margolin, Talovic and Weinstein, 1983), and the Family Environment Scale (Moos and Moos, 1981) are all well-validated questionnaires that have been used with problem drinker couples and families.

At the end of the assessment phase the therapist should be able to develop an integrated view of the problems that the individual excessive drinker and the family as a whole should address in the course of treatment. The results of the assessment should lead to a detailing of the major environmental, cognitive and emotional factors associated with the individual's drinking; a detailing of the ways (effective and ineffective) that the family have attempted to cope with the drinking; a detailing of the kinds of major problems that the family have; and an assessment of how the family function as a family unit, including strengths and weaknesses in communication and problem-solving. Given this comprehensive assessment the therapist can then make decisions about what problem areas require immediate intervention, who to involve in the treatment, and what kinds of treatment interventions might be most effective.

Gerry and Irene (McCrady, 1982) had been married 28 years when they sought outpatient treatment for Gerry's drinking. Gerry, 52, worked as a factory worker. Irene, 50, was a homemaker. They had five children, four of whom lived at home. Gerry had just been discharged from an alcohol detoxification programme, but had resumed daily drinking, consuming three to six drinks per day. Using the DACQ and self-monitoring cards for a week revealed three major areas related to his drinking: (1) environmental cues such as returning from work each day, sitting in his favourite chair at the kitchen table, and opening the refrigerator that they maintained for his and their sons' beers; (2) interpersonal situations in which he felt that he was not as good as other people, which elicited feelings of failure on his part; and (3) self-critical ruminations about interpersonal situations, as well as problems with his children, which led him to feel that he was a failure as a husband and father.

Irene had attempted to cope with Gerry's drinking in a variety of ways. Her responses on the SBQ showed that she had threatened to leave him, and told him that the children would lose respect for him. She also tried to stop his drinking by pouring alcohol down the sink, and by hiding it. She protected him from the consequences of his drinking by taking care of him when intoxicated, cleaning up after him when he drank, and getting him to bed. Both Gerry and Irene agreed that these actions were ineffective in stopping his drinking, and often led him to feel even more like drinking.

In the marital and family area, interviewing revealed that most of their children had had problems. Gerry and Irene had been involved in couples' counselling to learn how to handle children's problems, and felt that they were coping well with this area, even though they continued to feel concerned about their children and Gerry blamed himself for their problems. Structured questionnaires, including the Locke–Wallace Marital Adjustment Test and the Areas of Change Questionnaire, revealed that they had different perceptions of their relationship. Irene said that if she had her life to live over again she would not marry; Gerry said that he would marry the same person again. These differing perceptions seemed to reflect the depth of Irene's unhappiness with her life and her family. They both felt that they had problems in the financial and recreational area. Irene wished that Gerry would pay more attention to her, and participate in family decisions more, reflecting her general feeling that he was unavailable emotionally, and that there was a great deal of distance between them. Gerry reported being completely happy with Irene.

Gerry and Irene were asked to discuss a problem with each other, trying to solve it without therapist intervention. The therapist video-taped the interaction, and had it coded using the Marital Interaction Coding System. These observations revealed that Gerry and Irene had trouble discussing emotional issues, and that they misunderstood each other when either attempted to discuss their feelings. In addition, Irene tended to assume that she knew what Gerry was thinking, and was rarely corrected by Gerry, who would withdraw and sigh when he disagreed with Irene. Observations revealed that Irene often gave Gerry mini-lectures about his drinking and how to change it.

Putting all of this assessment material together led to a fairly specific treatment plan for Gerry and Irene. A number of individual issues had to be addressed including helping Gerry to stop drinking and learn ways to stay abstinent, and helping him learn to deal with his negative and self-critical thoughts and feelings. Irene needed to learn to cope differently with Gerry's drinking, especially by decreasing her lectures, letting him experience the negative consequences of drinking that occurred naturally, and learning to stop threatening him unless she was able to carry out these threats. Relationship treatment was designed to help the couple learn how to relate to each other on an emotional level, learn to work together to solve problems, and learn to spend positive time together again.

Treatment implications

The behavioural model directs treatment to multiple influences on alcohol consumption. Because of the broad focus, use of the model can guide the therapist's treatment decisions when relevant systems are unavailable. Thus, if the problem drinker will not participate in treatment, the model directs attention to what behaviours family members could focus upon in treatment. Conversely, if family members are unavailable or unwilling to participate in treatment, the model can direct the therapist's attention to the client's cognitive and behavioural responses to family cues, which could be modified even when the family member's behaviour could not. However, if all systems are potentially available, once interactions between these systems and drinking have been determined, treatment interventions are directed at systems which are believed to exert the greatest influence on drinking behaviour, and at systems which are the most important, though disrupted in their functioning.

Alcohol-focused interventions

We find it helpful to consider separately family interventions that are specifically focused around drinking and more general family problems. In the family area a number of interventions to modify alcohol-specific influences have been described (Hay, 1982; McCrady, 1982; Thomas and Santa, 1983). Such interventions have three major objectives: (1) to decrease family behaviours which may serve as antecedents to drinking; (2) to identify and change actions of family members which might be reinforcing drinking; (3) to increase the family's ability to support and reinforce positive changes in drinking.

A number of treatment procedures can be used to help family members change behaviours which trigger drinking. First, family members must realise that their well-intended attempts to prevent the drinker from drinking have the opposite effect. After having identified some of these behaviours through interviewing and using the SBQ, the therapist can ask family members to consider what has happened when they have nagged or attempted to get the drinker to stop. The excessive drinker can be asked about his/her reactions when the spouse does such things as hiding bottles or telling the drinker that drinking is bad for him/her. Usually, family members recognise that their attempts at control have been ineffective, but feel frustrated at not knowing how else to react. Feedback from the excessive drinker usually makes it clear that family control attempts have a negative impact, leading the drinker to want to drink more, and perhaps feel angry and guilty, rather than wanting to drink less.

If the family are unconvinced of the futility of trying to control the drinker, they can be encouraged to keep a journal or formal record of the ways that they are reacting to drinking. Such records may make it even clearer that their actions are ineffective.

Once the family are able to realise that they need to change, the therapist can help them brainstorm different ways to discuss their concerns about drinking. The entire family, including the excessive drinker, should be involved in this process. We usually suggest that family members follow several guidelines: (1) only discuss concerns when the excessive drinker is not drinking; (2) discuss their own feelings about the drinking, or a particular drinking situation, rather than lecturing the excessive drinker; and

(3) avoid blaming or criticising the excessive drinker. The excessive drinker should also be involved, by asking him/her for suggestions about what kinds of discussions about drinking would be most helpful/supportive. The entire family can then be helped to practise discussing concerns about drinking and drinking situations. Role-playing can be used with specific examples, and the therapist can give family members feedback, as well as ask them to discuss their feelings about this different way of discussing concerns about drinking.

Sometimes family members find it difficult to use these new skills in actual drinking situations. Asking them to practise at home can be helpful. In addition, the therapist may teach the partner some relaxation techniques, such as deep muscle relaxation or progressive muscle relaxation. Being able to relax can help the family member implement some of the skills being taught.

Meeting the second goal, changing behaviours which might be reinforcing drinking, can be accomplished in a similar manner. First, family members are helped to recognise the relationship between their actions and the maintenance of drinking. For example, the therapist can point out that providing orange juice and a backrub when the excessive drinker is hung over, and yelling when s/he is sober, may make drinking more desirable than abstinence. Similarly, the family can be helped to see that protecting the excessive drinker from painful consequences of drinking may also perpetuate the drinking cycle. Thus, the therapist may help the family think of different ways to act when the drinker is drinking. Guidelines suggested by the therapist include: (1) avoiding giving any positive attention to the excessive drinker when drinking; (2) allowing the naturally occurring negative consequences to unfold, even if they may be painful for the family to observe; (3) limiting their actions only to those that assure the physical safety of the excessive drinker. As described above, the entire family can brainstorm ideas about how to handle such situations, and they can be helped to role-play in the therapy session, and practise at home.

Irene was generally very protective of her husband. When he drank at a local bar he would often drive home, and then pass out in front of the house. Irene would go downstairs from their second-story apartment, rouse her husband, and half-carry, half-drag him upstairs, undress him and get him to bed. In discussing this sequence of events in therapy, the therapist questioned the necessity of bringing Gerry upstairs. Irene was concerned that he might be injured, and could not imagine just leaving him there. Gerry, however, said, 'That'd really shock me if I woke up in my car.' Irene, Gerry and the therapist agreed that it might help Gerry to be 'shocked', and they developed a plan with which Irene felt comfortable. Irene agreed that if Gerry came home intoxicated and passed out in the car, she'd go downstairs and check to reassure herself that he was not injured or ill. If it was not wintertime, then she'd return to their apartment and go to bed, leaving Gerry in the car. Since Gerry was not drinking at this point in the therapy, Irene did not have an opportunity to directly practise this plan. Instead, the therapist helped her to imagine this sequence of events, using a technique called covert rehearsal. Irene sat back in a comfortable chair, closed her eyes, and imagined the events as the therapist described each step in great detail. The therapist did this several times in the sessions, and asked Irene to practise this series of events in her imagination several times during the course of the week.

The third goal of alcohol-focused family interventions is to teach the family to provide positive reinforcement and support to the excessive drinker for not drinking. Many times the family do not express positive feelings about changes in drinking, feeling that the excessive drinker is 'doing what s/he should have done a long time ago'. The therapist can initiate a discussion of the value of positive feedback, and help the family to think of ways to express positive feelings about the drinker's successful attempts at change. They can practise giving the drinker feedback in the therapy session, and be asked to do so at home as well. In addition, it may be helpful for family members to provide concrete evidence of their support. This might take the form of a dish of ice cream, a note, or other form of positive appreciation. It is critical that the family recognise the difficulties inherent in initiating and sustaining changes in drinking, and learn the importance of their feedback.

The family can provide general support to the excessive drinker by discussing as a family how various alcohol-related issues should be handled. Examples include: whether or not to keep alcohol in the house, how to behave in situations where alcohol is served, and how to respond when the excessive drinker is experiencing some desire to drink. Too often, each family member may have his/her own notions about how to handle such situations. These individual notions lead to unilateral actions such as locking the liquor cabinet, or informing a hostess prior to a party that the partner cannot drink. Unilateral actions usually lead to anger, fights and resentment that may precipitate drinking episodes. If the family can come to mutual solutions about how to handle these problems, misunderstandings are avoided. As important, however, is that the family learn how to discuss and solve problems that concern them all.

Spouses and other family members may obtain help through professional or paraprofessional counsellors and therapists. If the excessive drinker is unwilling to get involved in the treatment, many of the interventions described above may be implemented without the excessive drinker present.

In addition, self-help groups are available for family members of excessive drinkers. The best known, Alanon, is for adult family members. The programme is modelled after the 12 Steps in Alcoholics Anonymous, and teaches family members that alcoholism (note that 'alcoholism' and 'alcoholic' are the terms used in Alanon, and therefore will be used in this discussion) is a disease which the family cannot control or change. Family members are taught that they are helpless to affect the drinker's actions, and that they have a disease as much as does the alcoholic. Alanon emphasises that the family member must learn to take care of him/herself, and attend to personal needs. Family members learn how to disengage from struggles around drinking, and are encouraged to build their own separate lives, even if they maintain their relationship with the excessive drinker. In the United States, comparable programmes, Alateen and Alatot (the latter being for pre-teenagers), are available for children of alcoholics. The children's programmes are usually sponsored by an Alanon member, and have an additional focus on helping the child realise that the parent's alcoholism is not the child's fault.

General family interventions

In directing interventions toward the family as a whole, no behavioural treatment programmes have been developed for whole families, so we will focus here on interventions for couples.

There are three major goals of interventions designed to help the couple make general changes in their relationship: (1) increase the overall level of positive interchange in the relationship; (2) teach communication skills which will both increase the positive value of the relationship and decrease the frequency of aversive and coercive interactions; (3) teach problem-solving and contracting skills to decrease the number of problem areas in the relationship, and hopefully decrease the number of antecedents to drinking.

To help couples become more positive with each other, several techniques may be used. The overall goal of these interventions is to help the couple enjoy each other more, and recall or re-experience some of the positive aspects of their relationship which they had lost through the years of excessive drinking. In addition, because spouses are asked to support the excessive drinker's attempts at change, it is most important that the spouse feel that he/she is receiving some consideration and caring from the excessive drinker, and that both are attending to their relationship.

To help couples increase positive aspects of their relationship, several homework assignments can be employed. For example, a 'caring day' (Stuart, 1980) might be assigned. During the treatment session, each partner develops a list of actions that their mate would enjoy during a particular day. These actions usually are small, such as making morning tea, putting an affectionate note in the partner's lunch, or massaging the partner's shoulders during the evening. Each spouse then selects one day during the week as his/her caring day, and does as many of these positive actions as possible that day. The receiving partner tries to notice positive actions each day during the week, and guesses which day was the caring day. This intervention has three positive effects: it helps each partner to note positive partner behaviours; it allows each partner to think about how to be giving rather than cruel to his/her mate; and it gives each partner the opportunity to enjoy receiving some kindness from the spouse.

Couples may also be instructed to identify a positive shared recreational activity to try during the week. As is evident from Steinglass's (1981) work, actively drinking families are dispersed, and spend little time together. The couple can be assisted in deliberately changing this state of affairs. The therapist must devote time to the task of planning an outing, by helping the couple think of a mutually desirable activity, and helping them plan when and how they will implement the outing. For couples who have spent little time together, initial outings might include the entire family, or might be rather short in duration and highly structured (such as going to a film). Structuring the assignment tends to decrease the chances of failure in such an assignment.

During the therapy hour, couples may be asked to think about characteristics of their partner which they find attractive or enjoyable, and can be asked to share these positive thoughts with the partner. All of these positively focused exercises are intended to increase the overall positive value of the relationship to the couple. Research on marital satisfaction (reviewed in Jacobson and Margolin, 1979) suggests that happy couples have a high rate of positive exchanges, and therapy efforts directed at increasing positive exchanges are associated with increased marital satisfaction.

Just helping couples be nice to each other is insufficient to make lasting changes in their relationships. Couples also need to learn better communication and problem-solving skills. There are a number of structured programmes to teach these skills, to which the reader can refer (e.g. Jacobson and Margolin, 1979), and these will therefore be reviewed here only briefly. Communication skills training should be tailored to the specific communication deficits which the therapist identified during the assessment phase of treatment. New skills are usually taught by describing the skill to the couple, showing them how to use it, and then having them practise the new skill, first in the therapy session and then at home. Examples of communication skills that can be taught include: reflective listening and paraphrasing; allowing the partner to finish speaking before beginning to speak; expressing appreciation of the importance of what the partner is saying, even if the other partner disagrees; expressing feelings directly; censoring negative and venomous remarks; staying on topic. It is clear that the list of communication skills is long, and deficits vary with the individual couple.

In addition to being able to communicate more clearly and empathically, couples also need to be able to identify and solve problems. Problem-solving training (Jacobson and Margolin, 1979) usually includes several steps: identifying the problem; collecting information relevant to the problem; brainstorming possible solutions to the problem; evaluating the pros and cons of the various solutions; selecting a solution for implementation; implementing the solution; evaluating the effectiveness of the solution. Couples are taught the steps in problem-solving in the therapy hour, and practise on simple problems first before attempting to solve major family problems. Once they can use the problem-solving strategy, they then can begin to apply it to more major problems.

RESEARCH EVIDENCE

Research has documented the importance of spouse involvement in treatment for drinking problems. Studies have consistently found that spouse involvement leads to a small but statistically significant increment in positive treatment outcomes (e.g. Hedburg and Campbell, 1974; McCrady, Paolino, Longabaugh and Rossi, 1979).

The authors' more recent research has focused on identifying the most important elements in spouse-involved outpatient treatment (McCrady, Noel, Abrams, Stout, Fisher-Nelson and Hay, 1986). In this research, different levels of intensity of spouse involvement have been compared. Couples seeking out-patient treatment for excessive drinking were randomly assigned to one of three levels of treatment intensity: minimal spouse involvement (MSI), alcohol-focused spouse involvement (AFSI), or alcohol-focused spouse involvement plus behavioural marital therapy (ABMT). All couples received 15 sessions of conjoint therapy, and were followed for 18 months after the completion of treatment.

Results of the study tended to favour the ABMT treatment approach. In this approach the excessive drinker was assisted in stopping drinking and learning how to maintain abstinence; the partner was assisted in learning how to cope with drinking and support abstinence; and the couple learned to improve communication and problem-solving skills. Couples in this treatment condition were more likely to complete treatment than MSI couples, and were more successful at decreasing their drinking than AFSI couples. During the first 6 months after treatment ABMT couples relapsed more slowly. Longer-term data analyses are preliminary, but suggest that ABMT couples continue on an improving course in their drinking and marital functioning, while MSI and AFSI couples are deteriorating in their drinking and marriages.

Taken as a whole, the research findings suggest that spouse involvement improves the likelihood of a positive outcome of treatment for excessive drinking. Our own research points to the importance of the kind of spouse involvement, and underscores the significance of helping couples change their relationship as well as their drinking. To date, such research has not been extended to whole families, suggesting areas for exciting investigation in the future.

SUMMARY AND CONCLUSIONS

Excessive drinking has profound consequences for the individual drinker and those that surround him or her. Family life is painful and disrupted, and families make a variety of efforts to cope with excessive drinking, some of them successful, some not. We have proposed a behavioural model for conceptualising drinking problems which systematically applies behavioural concepts across a range of intra-personal and interpersonal systems. It is our conviction that any model for understanding excessive drinking and modifying it must include

113

both of these levels of conceptualisation. A model of work with the individual without consideration of the social context of his or her drinking is as doomed to failure as is the rigid family model which ignores the multiple individual elements involved in excessive drinking.

REFERENCES

American Psychiatric Association (1980) *Diagnostic and statistical manual of mental disorders* (3rd edn), American Psychiatric Association, Washington, DC

Billings, A.G., Kessler, M., Gomberg, C.A. and Weiner, S. (1979) Marital conflict resolution of alcoholic and nonalcoholic couples during drinking and nondrinking sessions, *Journal of Studies on Alcohol, 40*, 183–95

Bohman, M., Sigvardsson, S. and Cloninger, C.R. (1981) Maternal inheritance of alcohol abuse, *Archives of General Psychiatry, 38*, 965–9

Cvitkovic, J.V. (1979) Alcohol use and communication congruence in alcoholic and nonalcoholic marriages. Doctoral dissertation, University of Pittsburg, 1978

Djukanovic, B., Milosavcevic, V. and Jovanovic, R. (1976) Drustveni zivot alkoholicaro i njihovih suprnga. (The social life of alcoholics and their wives.) *Alkoholizam, Beograd, 16*, 67–75 (From *Journal of Studies on Alcohol*, 1978, *39*, Abstract No. 1141)

Foy, D.W., Miller, P.M. and Eisler, R.M. (1975) The effects of alcohol consumption on the marital interactions of chronic alcoholics. Paper presented at Association for Advancement of Behavior Therapy, San Francisco

Frankenstein, W. (1982) Alcohol intoxication effects on alcoholics' marital interactions for three levels of conflict intensity. Unpublished Masters thesis, Rutgers University

Goodwin, D.W., Schulsinger, F., Hermanen, L., Guze, S. and Winokur, G. (1973) Alcohol problems in adoptees raised apart from alcoholic biological parents, *Archives of General Psychiatry, 28*, 238–43

Hay, W.M. (1982) The behavioral assessment and treatment of an alcoholic marriage: the case of Mr. & Mrs. L. In W.M. Hay and P.E. Nathan (eds), *Clinical case studies in the behavioral treatment of alcoholism*, Plenum, New York

Hedburg, A.G. and Campbell, L.A. (1974) A comparison of four behavioral treatments of alcoholism *Journal of Behavior Therapy and Experimental Psychiatry, 5*, 251–6

Hops, H., Wills, T.A., Patterson, G.R. and Weiss, R.L. (1971) *Marital interaction coding system* (Technical Report No. 8), Department of Psychology, Portland: University of Oregon

Jackson, J.K. (1954) The adjustment of the family to the crisis of alcoholism, *Quarterly Journal of Studies on Alcohol, 15*, 562–86

Jacobson, N. and Margolin, G. (1979) *Marital therapy*, Brunner/Mazel, New York

Johnson, V.E. (1973) *I'll quit tomorrow*, Harper and Row, New York

Klein, R.M. (1979) Interaction processes in alcoholic and nonalcoholic marital dyads. Doctoral dissertation, Washington University, 1978 (From *Journal of Studies on Alcohol, 40*, Abstract No. 169)

Locke, H.J. and Wallace, K.M. (1959) Short marital adjustment and prediction tests: their reliability and validity, *Marriage and Family Living, 21*, 251–5

McCrady, B.S. (1982) Conjoint behavioral treatment of an alcoholic and his spouse: the case of Mr. & Mrs. D. In W.M. Hay and P.E. Nathan (eds), *Clinical case studies in the behavioral treatment of alcoholism*, Plenum, New York

McCrady, B.S. (1985) Alcoholism. In D.H. Barlow (ed.), *Clinical handbook of psychological disorders: a step-by-step treatment manual*, Guilford Press, New York

McCrady, B.S., Paolino, T.J., Jr, Longabaugh, R. and Rossi, J. (1979). Effects on treatment outcome of joint admission and spouse involvement in treatment of hospitalized alcoholics, *Addictive Behaviors, 4*, 155–65

McCrady, B.S., Noel, N.E. Abrams, D.B., Stout, R., Fisher-Nelson, H. and Hay, W. (1986) Comparative effectiveness of three types of spouse involvement in outpatient behavioral alcoholism treatment, *Journal of Studies on Alcohol 47*, 459–67

Margolin, G., Talovic, S. and Weinstein, C.D. (1983) Areas of Change Questionnaire: a practical approach to marital assessment, *Journal of Consulting and Clinical Psychology, 51*, 920–31

Moos, R.H. and Moos, B.S. (1981) *Manual for the Family Environment Scale*, Consulting Psychologists Press, Palo Alto, CA

Orford, J., Guthrie, S., Nicholls, P., Oppenheimer, E., Egert, S. and Hensman, C. (1975) Self-reported coping behavior of wives of alcoholics and its association with drinking outcome, *Journal of Studies on Alcohol, 36*, 1254–67

Paolino, T.J., Jr and McCrady, B.S. (1977) *The alcoholic marriage: alternative perspectives*, Grune & Stratton, New York

Paolino, T.J., Jr. McCrady, B.S. and Diamond, S. (1978) Some alcoholic marriage statistics: an overview, *International Journal of the Addictions, 13*, 1285–93

Steinglass, P. (1979) The alcoholic family in the interaction laboratory, *Journal of Nervous and Mental Disease, 167*, 428–36

Steinglass, P. (1981) The alcoholic family at home. Patterns of interaction in dry, wet, and transitional stages of alcoholism, *Archives of General Psychiatry, 38*, 578–84

Stuart, R.B. (1980) *Helping couples change*, Guilford Press, New York

Thomas, E.J. and Santa, C.A. (1983) Unilateral family therapy for alcohol abuse: a working conception, *American Journal of Family Therapy, 10* 49–58

Vaillant, G. (1983) *The natural history of alcoholism. Causes, patterns and paths to recovery*, Harvard University Press, Cambridge MA

Wolin, S.J., Bennett, L.A. Noonan, D.L. and Teitelbaum, M. A. (1980) Disrupted family rituals: a factor in the intergenerational transmission of alcoholism, *Journal on Alcohol, 41*, 199–214

Zitter, R. and McCrady, B.S. (1979) The Drinking Antecedents and Consequences Questionnaire. Unpublished manuscript

6

Anorexia and the Family

Robert L. Palmer, Pamela Marshall and Rhoda Oppenheimer

Anorexia nervosa has come to be a widely known disorder but it remains poorly understood. To the detached outsider it can seem incomprehensible that so basic a process as eating can come to be disrupted in a way which threatens the well-being and even the life of otherwise healthy young people. The problem is deepened by questionable but widespread assertions that the disorder tends especially to afflict gifted and intelligent young women from privileged backgrounds. Why should 'good' girls from 'good' families end up in such a spiral of distress and suffering? The family confronted with the disorder in one of its members may similarly react with incomprehension and even bewilderment. Not uncommonly they feel some mixture of pity, anger, shame and guilt together with a feeling of impotence. Parents in particular may feel that they are to blame. What have they done wrong? Why has the simple matter of eating become so complex? Why has their daughter changed? Why is she doing it to them? Nowadays there is no shortage of answers to these questions. Newspapers, magazines, television and radio often make mention of anorexia nervosa and seek to explain it in terms of anything from an excess of advertising to a deficiency of zinc. The proposal that any one single idea can explain the complicated mess into which they and their daughter seem to have descended may be reassuring in the short term but on reflection is often experienced as being unsatisfactory, simplistic or even insulting. Dissatisfied with such journalistic views the family may seek out more extended and informed accounts. They may find a number of books by doctors and others which give an account of the disorder suitable for the general reader (Crisp, 1980, Palmer, 1980). Furthermore there are several autobiographical descriptions of anorexia nervosa which add their rich, albeit particular, perspective to the range of views on offer (Macleod,

1981; Wilkinson, 1984). Unfortunately these books by experts and former sufferers likewise tend to present a wide variety of explanations for the disorder. Families will not always emerge from their research less confused.

There are indeed many differences of view and emphasis in the literature about anorexia nervosa. Fortunately most professionals involved with the disorder would recognise a consensus view which emphasises the complex and multi-determined nature of its origin (Garfinkel and Garner, 1982). Biological, psychological and social ideas can all contribute to current understanding of the disorder. Different authors may emphasise particular factors but few would be sufficiently confident of their ground to wish to leave out other factors entirely. To take a narrow, one-sided or over-confident view is to leave the consensus and to risk being viewed as an eccentric or as a hobby-horse rider. However, in the matter of treatment, many clinicians may find it expedient to abandon their eclecticism in favour of enthusiasm for a particular treatment. Nevertheless the variety of treatment regimes on offer suggests that here, too, no one narrow answer has been found to be satisfactory. We will attempt to summarise, albeit in our own terms, something of this consensus concerning the nature of anorexia nervosa. In general, clinical eating disorders seem to arise when the issue of weight and eating control becomes entangled with wider personal issues in a way that proves to be unproductive and even disastrous. Most sufferers from anorexia nervosa enter the disorder via dietary restraint and weight loss arising from slimming for apparently commonplace reasons. Not surprisingly most sufferers are young women between the ages of 15 and 25. In common with other nutritionally deprived people the anorectic-to-be tends to be hungry, to be food-orientated, to be impulsive in her relationship to food and to experience a tendency towards excessive 'binge' eating if she fails to control herself. She may also be emotionally labile. Such are the common experiences of 'crash' dieters. Most sensibly give up the struggle in the face of these difficulties. However the anorectic continues; initially through a rewarding sense of self-control but increasingly because she fears the consequences of losing control. Her struggle becomes invested with meaning in terms of general self-evaluation. This increases her dread of loss of control. The individual's sense of self-worth and emotional stability thus become almost entirely dependent upon the struggle for control of weight and eating. Entanglement between these two sets of issues may occur more readily in young women of obsessional personality and in those coming from backgrounds in which issues of personal control are especially valued or identified with physical or nutritional matters. Home circumstances in which 'rocking the boat' seems especially dangerous may likewise contribute to the anorectic's failure to relinquish her position of tight control. Changes occurring in the family and in the biology of the individual as a consequence of the developing illness may themselves act as further perpetuating factors. Before long the individual sufferer finds herself at an abnormally low weight, showing various physical changes including amenorrhoea, and fearfully concerned about avoiding weight gain. She has thus come to fulfil the diagnostic criteria for anorexia nervosa. She finds herself increasingly cut off from the normal preoccupations of her peers. If she is to recover she has to restore her weight and eating towards a normal pattern and also change psychologically. Most treatment regimes seek to help the anorectic by providing some measure of prescription and supervision for the first task and some kind of psychotherapy for the second.

Anorexia nervosa of a classic and severe kind can be a devastating and even life-threatening disorder. In terms of definition the picture is complicated in two ways (Palmer, 1982). Firstly, mild degrees of entanglement between weight and eating and personal issues are not unusual, and therefore what might be described as subclinical anorexia nervosa is relatively common in young women. Furthermore, dips into disorder which are severe in terms of weight loss may, nevertheless, be brief and not go on to the chronic disorder which is common in the clinic. Secondly, the tendency towards binge eating, which is present in most starved populations, may come to be an important feature of low-weight anorexia nervosa. Here it is characteristically accompanied by abnormal weight control methods such as self-induced vomiting or laxative abuse. Such bulimic anorectics sometimes gain weight but may become stuck in a new morbid position which is dominated by extreme binge eating at a normal weight. Other individuals may come to this position without ever having fulfilled the criteria for anorexia nervosa. This state is known as bulimia nervosa or simply as bulimia. These syndromes may be long-lived and disruptive for the sufferer, but may also occur in mild and short-lived forms. The literature on eating disorders does not always differentiate sufficiently between anorexia nervosa, bulimia nervosa and their milder variants. Most writings and ideas are derived from the study of subjects with the classical disorder of abstinent anorexia nervosa in its most severe form. In this respect this chapter will be no exception, in that we will mainly address ourselves to family issues relevant to the origins, course and care of the anorectic subject. We believe,

119

however, that many of the same principles are likely to apply to other similar eating disorders.

THE FAMILY AND THE ORIGIN OF ANOREXIA NERVOSA

A family pondering its possible contribution to the origins of anorexia nervosa in a member is likely to think in the main of the way in which the interplay of relationships within the family may have upset the sufferer and somehow led to her illness. Likewise the professional literature on the subject tends to a similar emphasis. However in the broad sense the family can also contribute by means of the genetic endowment which they contribute, or by being the instrument of a particular kind of socialisation. We will discuss each of these aspects in turn.

Genetic factors

There is at present no definitive answer to the question as to whether there is any specific genetic component in the aetiology of anorexia nervosa. The apparently changeable prevalence of the disorder over recent times, and evidence of its sensitivity to cultural pressure, would tend to suggest that a genetic factor is unlikely to be of great importance. However it could be that a specific genotype might convey a vulnerability which becomes manifest only under certain environmental circumstances. Alternatively, the vulnerability could be of a non-specific kind which might find different expression under other conditions.

The role of a genetic component in any illness may be studied by an examination of the prevalence of the disorder in first-degree relatives of the affected person, by twin studies comparing the concordance rate between monozygotic and dizygotic (i.e. identical and non-identical) twins, by means of adoption studies and by seeking genetic markers. Only the first two methods have been used in anorexia nervosa, and those studies that have been carried out have been relatively few and on a small scale. Studies of first-degree relatives have suggested that there may be some excess of definable eating disorder in the families of anorectic subjects. Thus Theander (1970) suggests that the siblings of an anorectic have a 7 per cent risk of developing the disorder. This is clearly above the general expectation. Likewise Crisp (1980) reports that some 14 per cent of

mothers and 9 per cent of fathers had a history which was consistent with either marginal or frank anorexia nervosa. The biggest twin study to date is that of Crisp, Hall and Holland (1985), who reported a similar concordance rate for dizygotic twins as for non-twin siblings. However they report a 55 per cent concordance rate for monozygotic (identical) twins. This difference is highly suggestive of a specific genetic component but in the absence of adoption studies these data are not conclusive. Identical twins may well have had almost identical treatment during childhood. The authors of the study argue that the special bond between identical twins may be threatened at puberty and a joint regression into anorexia nervosa could be a means of preserving the partnership. However, there seems at present to be no evidence that twins as such are more prone to the disorder. Nevertheless, shared environment remains an important possible explanation for the familial nature of the disorder in general. Anorexia nervosa in siblings may reflect a common response to environmental difficulty, or when it occurs sequentially could perhaps be seen as an attempt to maintain family homeostasis (Crisp and Toms, 1972).Crisp et al. (1985) quote the case of an adopted family in which there were three biologically unrelated members, all of whom developed anorexia nervosa. This is a powerful anecdote. Clearly in such a case environment is likely to have played a very important role in the development of the disorder.

There are similar problems of interpretation of data which suggest that families containing an anorectic may also contain more than their fair share of affective disorder (Winokur, March and Mendels, 1980) and of alcohol problems (Halmi and Loney, 1973). Perhaps the parents of anorectics pass on a non-specific genetic vulnerability which may manifest itself as anorexia nervosa. However it is at least equally plausible that the relationship with a depressive parent or with a parent with an alcohol problem may promote the development of the disorder in the offspring by non-genetic means.

Family as agent of socialisation

The family is an important agent of socialisation for the offspring. In addition to passing on a genetic endowment and providing a particular environment of personal relationships the family conveys to its children a version of the attitudes, values and expectations of the wider culture. This version will be a selection determined both by the sub-group to which the family belongs and also by the particular characteristics of the senior family members.

Unfortunately, most of the evidence upon which generalisations could be made is anecdotal, or at best based upon uncontrolled clinical series. Until recently there has been some evidence that anorexia nervosa occurs particularly in families rated as belonging to the higher social classes. However, this tendency has been less marked or absent in recent studies, and it could be that earlier reports were subject to a selection bias. There have also been repeated reports that parents of anorectic subjects are older than would be expected on average. There seems to be no consistent size of sibship or birth order. It has been speculated that the combination of older parents drawn from the middle or upper classes may mean that typical parents of an anorectic are people who have postponed procreation until they have successfully established themselves in other spheres, and who may be inclined to pass on a rather rigid and success-orientated version of the wider society's expectations.

Some writers have suggested that the families of anorectic patients have a greater than average preoccupation with weight, eating, health or exercise, and that such a preoccupation antedates the onset of the disorder of the family member (Kalucy, Crisp and Harding, 1977). Such families might be expected to hand on to their children an especially strong 'dose' of the culture's preconceptions and beliefs about these issues. Many professionals working with eating-disordered subjects are impressed by the numbers of parents who are either personally or professionaly highly involved with such topics. It seems that many families contain a doctor, a dietician, a restaurateur or an athlete. However, such impressions are based upon uncontrolled observation. Nevertheless it certainly makes sense if families in which weight and eating are already invested with a greater meaning produce more than their fair share of anorectic daughters or even sons. Despite anecdotal reports to the contrary parental obesity does not seem to be a characteristic of anorexia nervosa (Halmi, Strauss and Goldberg, 1978). Such issues as vegetarianism or unusual food beliefs have not been studied systematically.

Clinical impressions suggest that the 'typical' family in which there is an anorectic member may be one in which emotional control is highly prized and where communication, particularly of negative emotion, is discouraged. Furthermore discussion of difficult topics, for instance sexuality, may be not only avoided, but actually deemed to be inappropriate. Such a family style may contribute to the negative sexual attitudes which are characteristic of eating-disordered subjects. These characteristics are best discussed in the context of more ambitious dynamic and family models.

Dynamic and interpersonal factors

There are several essentially psychodynamic models which attempt to explain the development of anorexia nervosa. Earlier models tend to concentrate heavily on a single aspect of the disorder. A frequent focus is the anorectic's fear of her own sexual impulses. These models suggest that anorexia nervosa is a means of controlling fears about sexuality. This is achieved by replacing sexual fears with fears about body size, as the latter are more easily controlled. Such views have been criticised for being unduly narrow. Other models acknowledge the importance of sexuality in the development of the disorder, but set it in a broader context. The views of two important writers on anorexia nervosa, namely Arthur Crisp of London and the late Hilde Bruch from the USA, will be examined in some detail.

Crisp postulates that anorexia nervosa may be seen as an avoidance of psychosexual maturity, and that this basic avoidance manifests itself in a secondary avoidance of a normal body weight. Pubertal body weight is viewed as a threshold which presents the individual with the problems of sexuality, autonomy and separation. The pre-anorectic individual is seen as someone who is ill-equipped to deal with the demands of adolescence and who copes by avoiding them through reducing her body weight and regressing to a pre-pubertal state. This regression is said to offer a simpler existence, a sense of renewed control and, paradoxically, greater autonomy, albeit within a narrower range. Crisp attributes the anorectic's failure to cope to a number of factors including aspects of family functioning. Thus the changes of adolescence may pose a threat to other members of the family as well as to the individual herself. For instance the child growing up may re-awaken the mother's own adolescent problems; evidence of the child's sexuality may exacerbate the mother's own sexual fears; or the child who is seen as a means of fulfilling her parents' unrealised expectations may threaten their stability if she appears to be pursuing her own. It may be seen that in some ways the child/anorectic fulfils a purpose within the family. Crisp is anxious to point out, however, that a combination of factors are required for the development of anorexia nervosa, and that disturbed family functioning is only one of the forces involved.

Hilde Bruch (1973) shares the view that several factors may contribute to the development of anorexia nervosa, and agrees that the disorder may be seen as a maladaptive means of achieving autonomy and control. She places emphasis on the mother–child relationship and suggests that a faulty relationship plays an important role in the development of the disorder. She proposes that the mother's responses are absent, contradictory or inadequate, and thus confuse the child to the point where she is unable to differentiate between her emotional and nutritional needs. This may result in her mixing up feelings, such as hunger and upset, so that she equates control of her hunger with emotional control. This inability to disentangle emotional and physiological needs may make the child over-dependent on the emotional responses of others to let her know what she is feeling and how she should respond. Such a situation makes an independent existence seem particularly difficult and threatening. In addition it is suggested that the child finds it difficult to separate from her parents because she is somehow indebted to them. Bruch describes families with anorectic members as being characterised by a spirit of parental sacrifice with both parents being in competition to suffer most for the child. This places an obligation on the child to live up to her parents' expectations and satisfy their demands. These demands may prohibit adolescent rebellion because they necessitate high standards of achievement, morality and success. Both Crisp and Bruch find an important role for family factors in their models of the genesis of anorexia nervosa, but they also clearly emphasise individual vulnerability. This is important since it tempers their accounts of pathological mothering and family disturbance which might otherwise all too easily contribute to a scapegoating of the parents as the simple causes of the disorder.

Other writers have laid even more emphasis upon the role of the family in anorexia nervosa, and speculate that the disorder may serve a function within a disordered family system. Such models suggest that the anorectic child plays an important role in maintaining family homeostasis. They take the view that the family operates as a system and is regulated by boundaries which are determined by the transactional patterns between its members. Whilst each family is seen as having certain preferred patterns of functioning circumstances often demand that these are adapted and restructured. It is suggested that the strength of the family system depends on its ability to adapt to stress. The preferred manner is one which maintains continuity but permits restructuring. Some families may respond to stress by sticking rigidly to existing transactional patterns. This lack of flexibility is thought to generate dysfunctional patterns, including eating disorders. Key examples of such views have been contributed by

Selvini-Palazzoli and by Minuchin. Both Palazzoli's group (Milan) (Palazzoli, 1974) and Minuchin's group (Philadelphia) (Minuchin, Rosman and Baker, 1978) have suggested that anorexia nervosa may be viewed as an expression of family dysfunction.

The Milan group adopted an approach based on Haley's model of family systems (Haley, 1959). Like Crisp and Bruch, they identify the anorectic child as occupying a role in maintaining marital unity. Palazzoli suggests that a series of secret rules and alliances operate between the family members. Frequently this may involve an alliance where the child is forced to side with each parent against the other. Within this role the child is encouraged to make up for the other partner's shortcomings. This 'three-way matrimony' achieves a false sense of solidarity, but places the child in an almost impossible situation. She is required to divide her sympathy equally between both parents by playing the secret role of both husband and wife at once. Such systems may operate fairly well until threatened by changes, such as adolesence. It is then that anorectic symptoms may occur as a means of maintaining the balance. The disturbed marital relationship which necessitates such alliances is characterised by 'a façade of respectability and unity' concealing a sense of 'deep disillusionment'. The need for respectability prohibits the involvement of others outside the family, and requires a search for some kind of resolution within the family. Both parents compete for moral superiority through self-sacrifice. They both wish to appear the more persecuted of the pair. The child occupies a complex position where each parent seeks her support in secret but does not do so openly, since that would deny them the role of the victim.

Minuchin's group addresses similar issues. They suggest that the development of a psychosomatic illness in a child is related to three factors — a special type of family organisation and functioning, the involvement of the child in parental conflict and a physiological vulnerability, although they question the presence of this last in anorexia nervosa.

Their view is that the functioning of such families may be characterised by enmeshment, over-protectiveness, rigidity and lack of conflict resolution. Members of enmeshed families are over-involved and over-responsive to each other, and intrude on each other's thoughts and feelings. The roles of individuals are unclear and personal autonomy is severely hampered. A family system characterised by over-protectiveness is similarly restricting. Increased concern for the welfare of others results in protective responses being consistently sought and supplied. Thus when one member of the family is sick all become involved. Overt individual protest is inhibited and indirect expression becomes the only means of conveying personal wishes to others. A pattern of rigidity is demonstrated by an unwillingness to accept any change within the family and a rigid maintenance of preferred transactional patterns. The existence of conflict tends to be denied, or the manner in which it is dealt with is inconsistent. Issues are not negotiated or resolved. The sick child may help the family to avoid conflict by becoming a common focus of concern. In turn the family may reinforce her anorectic behaviour in order to preserve the pattern of conflict avoidance.

There are obvious similarities between the observations of the Milan and Philadelphia groups, in particular the involvement of the child in parental conflict, the presence of secret alliances and the over-involvement of family members. Unfortunately such matters are difficult to study using other than clinical and descriptive methods, and these family theories are supported by little objective evidence. Crisp, Harding and McGuinness (1974) studied the psychoneurotic status of parents before and after their daughters' in-patient weight restoration and demonstrated an increase in parental psychopathology after their daughters' weight had been restored. This lends support to the idea that the illness is protective of one or both members of the parental pair. However, in general attempts to demonstrate objective differences between anorectic and control families have been unimpressive in their results. The present authors have recently studied the responses of a series of anorectic patients to a self-report questionnaire, the Parental Bonding Instrument (PBI). This systematically, albeit briefly, seeks the subjects' recollections of their parents' behaviour during their childhood up to the age of 16 years. The results did not tend to confirm the presence of predicted patterns of parental relationships and the most impressive finding was the variety of parental styles which were reported (Palmer, Oppenheimer and Marshall, 1984).

Summary

Families do seem to be involved in the causation of anorexia nervosa. This must be the provisional conclusion from the large quantity of observations which support such a view. However, the predominantly anecdotal quality of the observations means that it is proper to preserve a measure of scepticism, especially about the value of particular detailed formulations. What then should be the attitude of a family to their own possible role in the anorectic disorder of a family member? Certainly it would seem important to discourage an attitude of excessive blame or breast-beating. At the same time the family need to accept that their own current and future attitudes and behaviour may importantly affect the process and outcome of the disorder in the sick family member. Their willingness to be open-minded and to change themselves may not be sufficient to divert the course of established anorexia nervosa but it often seems to be a necessary condition if change is to occur. Thus, for instance, the rather socially diffident daughter of an anxious mother was seen as having developed anorexia nervosa as a retreat, after a failed attempt to grow up and establish an independent life. The disorder emerged out of slimming, which itself seemed to represent an attempt to improve her social acceptability and self-esteem. Once established the retreat also proved rewarding for the mother, in that it substituted for the lack of support of her husband whose own life revolved around football refereeing and other 'male' pursuits. Mother and daughter became inseparable companions in a limited but protective life. Each was aware both of the comforts and drawbacks of the situation, in particular the stuck state of the daughter's development. Whilst the father too was worried, he was perhaps also relieved of any sense of guilt at neglecting his wife. For recovery to occur it was helpful for both parents to relieve their daughter of her sense of respons-ibility for their happiness and well-being. This, although perhaps unconsciously acquired, was nevertheless experienced as a burden and a worry. Only then could she clearly tackle her own problems of lack of self-confidence and poor social skills. In this case, although it is possible to see the parents as involved in the promotion of the illness, a concept such as 'blame' seems quite inappropriate. This is usually the case. Professionals involved in helping anorectics and their families need themselves to avoid both dogmatism and scapegoating in their attempts to apply their theories of family involvement in the disorder. Otherwise there is a danger of merely adding their own rigidity to the system of beliefs which entraps the sufferer.

THE FAMILY IN AND AROUND TREATMENT

Presentation to care

The process by which individuals with eating disorders present to professional agencies for help has received little formal study. However it is clear that some anorectic and bulimic subjects do not present. Many of these have severe disorder. This is probably especially so for bulimia, although some severe low-weight anorectics also avoid contact with professional services. The family is often involved in presentation of eating-disorder subjects, especially those at low weight. Such subjects may express their ambivalence about change by failing to seek help themselves but allowing others to cajole them to do so.

If anorexia nervosa is construed as an aspect of a family system which has thereby sought to preserve its stability, it would follow that forces within the family might well tend to delay or prevent presentation of the anorectic to treatment. Certainly professionals often report cases where the family seems to have colluded with the anorectic in doing nothing about a state of disorder which seems evident and extreme to an outsider. However, many forces may be at work in such a situation, and these need to be explored with delicacy and tact when presentation finally occurs. The patient and her family may be very wary of the stigma involved in presentation, especially to a psychiatrist. In addition the family may fear that they could be blamed for the disorder. Parents may be tantalised by the apparent simplicity of the remedy for their daughter's state. They may feel that all she needs to do is to start eating sensibly and all will be well. They may be slow to give up hope that their encouragement or nagging will have the desired effect if they persist just a little longer. Furthermore, because the issue seems so simple the family may feel that others are unlikely to meet with more success than they. Lastly, they may fear that by seeking professional help the issue will become emotionally more complicated for them.

Eating-disorder clinics also on occasion receive referrals of young women propelled along by their family who are not suffering an eating disorder and whose preoccupation with weight and eating is only a little excessive. Here parental concern may have led to the worried over-extension of the concept of anorexia nervosa to include commonplace dieting or food fads. Parents assume these to be the herald of the severe disorder which they may have read about in the newspapers. Sometimes such a presentation represents little more than parental panic, which readily disperses with reassurance. In other cases it may be part of a persistent pattern of over-concern which itself warrants attention.

A further pattern of presentation involves the individual or her family in seeking help for only a part of the problem. Thus concern may centre around the issue of amenorrhoea or weight loss without the patient's abnormal attitudes being acknowledged or explored. Again a kind of collusion may be present whereby both the patient and her family are willing to seek help around the physical symptom alone and thereby avoid wider and more painful attention.

Access to the health services generally occurs via the general practitioner. Even when the diagnosis of anorexia nervosa is agreed, the issue of whether, and to whom, he should refer a case for specialist assessment and treatment may be importantly influenced by such issues. Certainly anorexia nervosa is usually construed as a psychiatric problem, but nevertheless its physical manifestations and complications may make presentation to a general physician seem rational. Indeed many general physicians see and manage anorectic patients without reference to any form of psychological help. It is arguable that such referrals reflect the desire of the patient, and often the family, to play down the psychological aspects of the disorder. Conversely referral to a non-medical therapist working alone may reflect a desire to avoid the essential issues of weight gain and physical change. Helpers in the field need to address both issues.

A number of voluntary self-help groups have arisen out of the felt need of eating-disordered people and their families for support and sharing of their difficulties with others in similar situations. The Norwich-based Anorexia Family Aid provides not only a local support group but a nationally available information service about help of all kinds for eating-disordered people (address: Sackville Place, 44 Magdalen Street, Norwich, Norfolk NR3 1JE; Telephone 0603 621414). Anorexia Aid has local groups in various parts of the country, although its activities and strength seem to vary widely from place to place.

Engaging in treatment

When the anorectic and her family have reached an appropriate specialist they must all embark on the delicate matter of engaging in treatment. For professionals who deal with many such patients this would be a familiar process, but for the patient it is always a worrying and frightening affair. She will be ambivalent about treatment and the prospect of change. The management of this ambivalence is of crucial importance in the process of engagement. For the family it is an anxious time, and a doctor or other therapist who is inexperienced in this particular task may share this anxiety. Often the key to success is to avoid entering into any kind of battle with the patient, but rather to achieve some shared understanding of her situation which acknowledges her mixed feelings. This will be achieved only by detailed assessment and the careful establishment of a relationship which allows the patient to consider the possibility of change. She must contain the battle of her own mixed feelings within herself and be helped with it rather than allowing those around her to take over one side of the battle leaving her free simply to resist. Often by the time of presentation such battle lines have been drawn up within the family, but the therapist must avoid the tempting option of joining the parents' side. Likewise if the therapist provokes a battle against the patient the family may well join in robustly on either side, but in every case the patient will lose out. Not uncommonly a situation develops in which detention under a section of the Mental Health Act is threatened or even evoked, and once again the family would be involved. In practice such compulsory treatment is seldom justified, and may merely increase the determination of the patient to resist. For this variety of reasons it is usually advantageous to involve the family in the initial process of assessing the problem and engaging the patient. The therapist should take pains to establish an appropriate rapport with them, although this should never be at the expense of the relationship with the patient.

At many centres the parents, spouse or other family member would be seen at the initial appointment, both jointly with the patient and separately. This initial contact can be used to give information to the family, collect information from the family, begin to establish a working relationship with the family and even to open up discussion of relevant emotional issues which will be developed in later individual and family therapy. This first contact may be crucial. There should be a clear opportunity for both patient and family to express their reservations about the prospect of treatment as well as their hopes.

There is no one optimal method of conducting such first contact and assessment. We will describe our own practice as an example. The patient is invited to attend an extended out-patient appointment which lasts about 2 hours. She is requested to bring with her a member or members of her family or others who are close to her. Thus a patient attending with her parents will initially be seen for 10 minutes or so by both the psychiatrist and social worker, together with her family. This gives all parties the opportunity to state their initial position, in each other's presence, before having a more prolonged and private interview with one of the professionals. Typically the psychiatrist will see the patient whilst the social worker interviews the family.

Our method of collecting information from the family is based on the use of a family tree or geneogram (Lieberman, 1980). The geneogram is drawn up on a large sheet of paper, during the interview, and will consist of information on family members including grandparents and beyond if appropriate. Information is collected and shared about the personal and environmental resources through which the family has maintained and passed on its identity and culture from one generation to the next. This will include views on practices, careers, achievements, behaviours and beliefs, secrets, family styles and language, ways of expressing emotion and methods of dealing with sex education and so on. Facts are recorded about family members' height, weight and health in addition to the developmental history of the patient herself. A geneogram can aid in defining and understanding difficult or 'no-go' areas for family discussion. Sometimes the construction of the geneogram may itself initiate some change in understanding for the family members themselves, as well as providing useful information for the treatment team. Such information can be both enhanced and utilised in later therapy.

The first assessment meeting and the construction of the geneogram provides an important beginning in understanding, and usually ends in the construction of preliminary hypotheses or 'stories' about the psychosocial underpinnings of the disorder, especially when it is put together with the information collected from the patient herself. In our clinic the psychiatrist and social worker talk together after the individual interviews and before meeting the patient again for further discussion and to make a treatment offer. It is the patient's choice whether or not she wishes her parents or others to be involved in this last part of the first meeting. In general we try to adopt a style which encourages openness but respects and seeks to define 'secrets' between family members. Although we are impressed by the variety rather than the uniformity of the interactions in families containing an anorectic member, it does seem to be the case that such 'secrets' and communication deficits are frequently present and seem to be of some importance. Not uncommonly such problems arise around the topic of sexuality, where there may be an atmosphere of embarrassment, secrecy and taboo. Eating-disordered subjects have often had adverse sexual experiences, sometimes involving childhood sexual abuse. These experiences may have been dealt with in a way which creates increased difficulty for the patient (Oppenheimer, Howells, Palmer and Chaloner, 1985).

Family involvement in treatment

Recovery from anorexia nervosa involves two complementary tasks. Firstly there is the task of restoring weight and eating to a more normal level and pattern. Secondly there is the task of promoting psychological and perhaps interpersonal change. Typically the family will have been involved prior to presentation in an attempt to help the patient with the task of weight restoration. Characteristically their efforts will not have been successful. Most treatment regimes seek to remove this task from the family and place responsibility back with the patient. In many cases this may require the patient to seek other help and supervision by becoming a hospital in-patient and accepting nursing care. Even very early accounts of the disorder, such as that of Sir William Gull (1874), suggest that the parents' capacity to change their daughter's eating may have been exhausted by the time she is seen by a doctor. Others may be in a better position to help. Nevertheless ultimately the patient must feed herself. Because she is hungry she will be prepared to do this provided she can be made to feel sufficiently safe. The family can contribute to this sense of safety by acknowledging her fear of overeating and by being prepared to help set appropriate limits for her. Unfortunately families will often add their own urgings to the anorectic's drive to eat and thereby create a situation which is even more fearful for her. To someone struggling with an appetite which is experienced as potentially out of control, it is not helpful to be repeatedly tempted with 'favourite' foods. The need is rather to create an atmosphere of expectation that food is eaten in the normal way with upper as well as lower limits. It is not obvious to the family that an anorectic member may want reassurance that she will be prevented from overeating, particularly when she has given no indication to them that this is what she fears most. Firm encouragement to eat a normal meal, combined with sympathetic acknowledgement of this fear, is certainly the best way of trying to help the anorectic to eat more. Simple explanation of such matters may help the family to cope with and avoid difficult mealtime scenes. Such combinations of clear expectation and supervision are the backbone of most in-patient treatment regimes, and have on the whole taken the place of complex behavioural programmes.

Probably a majority of low-weight anorectics receive hospital treatment at some stage, although only a small minority of bulimics require such treatment. When an anorectic is admitted to a specialist unit it would be characteristic that the matter of eating and weight gain would quickly become under appropriate control. Even this 'success' can be difficult and emotionally complex for the family. They may feel relief, but at the same time they may feel jealousy, guilt or anger that strangers have succeeded where they have failed. Such emotional reasons or misunderstandings may lead them to interfere with the treatment or collude with their daughter's desire to resist treatment. It has recently been demonstrated that aspects of the family's emotional state may be predictive of early drop-out from treatment. In particular, high expressed emotion (EE), and especially critical comments measured in a standard way, were associated with drop-out (Szmuckler, Eisler, Russell and Dare, 1985). However, such problems can usually be avoided, or at least put in their proper perspective, by regular contact between the treatment team and the family. This contact may take the form both of informal conversations and formal family meetings. Such meetings may perform a variety of functions, including actual therapy of the family system. At the least they provide an avenue of communication between patient, family and treating professionals which can be used to avoid the more troublesome misunderstandings and differences of opinion. Again our own practice may be neither optimal nor typical, but serves as an example of one way of addressing such issues. Every 3 or 4 weeks throughout the anorectic's in-patient stay, and sometimes beyond, the whole family is invited to meet with key members of the treatment team — typically the consultant, the social worker and the individual therapist who may be either a junior doctor or a nurse. The family will have agreed to attend these meetings as part of the initial treatment contract with the patient. Three or four staff members meeting with a family may result in a group of up to a dozen people, but the style of the meeting aims to model openness, frankness and honesty and to avoid the kind of splitting, manipulation and masked communication which might otherwise be characteristic of these families in times of trouble. It will tend to become evident in such meetings if families actively avoid or seek to divert attention from important problem areas. The patient may need to come to terms with the difficulty which the family has in dealing with some issues, and it may be helpful for her to recognise that at least part of the problem is not hers alone. Family meetings are used to share information and

133

feelings about the current treatment situation, about the patient's disorder and most importantly about the emotional context and issues which have contributed to its origins and perpetuation. Often the meetings seem to promote both shared understanding and change. They may be construed as a form of family therapy used as an adjunct to the other treatments.

Family therapy

Family therapy has been widely advocated as an appropriate treatment for anorexia nervosa. It may be used as a principal psychotherapeutic approach to what we have described as the second task of recovery — namely, promoting psychological and interpersonal change. However, it has been advocated as the sole intervention in some cases, and here the issues of the first task, namely weight and eating, may also be addressed directly in the family group. Typically this has been suggested as appropriate where the patient is a child still living within, and subject to the care of, the family of origin. Here the task of getting their child to eat may be placed fairly and squarely upon the parents and even enacted within the family meeting. Indeed some family therapists have incorporated the notion of a family therapy lunch session as an integral part of their treatment (Minuchin, 1974). More usually, family therapy is concerned with addressing issues relevant to the second task. Here it may be used as the sole form of psychotherapy or as an adjunct to individual therapy. Many authorities would agree with Garfinkel and Garner (1982), who suggest that when the patient is aged 16 or younger, and living at home, family therapy should usually be the primary mode of psychotherapy. Such therapy seeks to promote change in the over-rigid and enmeshed patterns of relationship which are often seen in these families. Different therapists advocate different styles. Many therapists seek to promote room to manoeuvre by freeing communication and clarifying patterns of relationship. Others, having developed a hypothesis of the family structure, seek to change it by interventions or injunctions which do not necessarily involve promotion of shared understanding of the problem. Therapists may use paradoxical statements or injunctions to try to change interactional patterns thought to be important in perpetuating the disorder. An example for consideration is one in which the mother, perhaps for her own reasons, appears to be notably over-concerned and controlling of her daughter in a way which excludes the father and prevents him from acting appropriately. Such a mother might be congratulated for taking on so much of her husband's role, thereby allowing him to pursue his own life and interests in a way that she cannot. She might be encouraged to carry on with this notable sacrifice for the sake of her husband. The aim of such an intervention would be to lead her to question herself, and perhaps to feel that she is missing out and letting her husband off lightly. She might then seek to change her position in a way which would not have been likely had the 'self-sacrifice' been seen as for the sake of the daughter. The covert purpose would be to relieve the daughter and allow the father more influence.

At present whilst there are many rich clinical accounts of family therapy with eating-disordered patients there is little other than clinical wisdom and tradition to suggest which technique is best in which situation. However a major trial of individual versus family treatment of anorexia nervosa after in-patient weight restoration is currently in progress at the Maudsley Hospital, London. It is hoped that this study may throw some light on the appropriate place of family therapy. Meanwhile, its use as a central mode of therapy in younger patients and as adjunct in older patients would seem to be sensible. However, for some patients the issue of successful separation from their family of origin may be the appropriate aim in therapy, and for a few of these the actual involvement of the family may not be helpful. For others the relevant 'family' group at the time of treatment may sometimes be the family of marriage. The pattern of difficult relationships and the changes necessary for recovery within a marriage involving an anorectic subject may be as important and as problematic as are the changes within the family of origin.

CONCLUSION

Anorexia nervosa is a complex disorder, and family relationships seem to be of some importance in its promotion and in its therapy. Furthermore, although it is possible to construe the disorder as reflecting family trouble, and even as contributing to family homeostasis, there is no doubt that the occurrence of anorexia nervosa within a family also constitutes a new trouble, and a potential multiplier of distress and possible disaster. It is always difficult to be confident about what is cause and what is effect. Therapists who are involved with an anorectic member owe them a skilful and detached assessment, a knowledgeable if sceptical use of theory and decisive offers of robust intervention. They also owe, to the patient and to her family, respect, concern and care when they intervene in painful areas.

REFERENCES

Bruch, H. (1973) *Eating disorders: obesity, anorexia nervosa and the person within*, Basic Books, New York

Crisp, A.H. (1980) *Anorexia nervosa: let me be*, Academic Press, London

Crisp, A.H. and Toms, D.A. (1972) Primary anorexia nervosa or weight phobia in the male. Report on 13 cases, *British Medical Journal, 1*, 334–8

Crisp, A.H., Harding, B. and McGuinness, B. (1974) Anorexia nervosa: psychoneurotic characteristics of parents: relationship to prognosis. A quantitative study, *Journal of Psychosomatic Research, 18*, 167–73

Crisp, A.H., Hall, A. and Holland, A.J. (1985) Nature and nurture in anorexia nervosa: a study of 34 pairs of twins, one pair of triplets, and an adoptive family, *International Journal of Eating Disorders, 4*, 5–27

Garfinkel, P.E. and Garner, D.M. (1982) *Anorexia nervosa: a multidimensional perespective*, Brunner/Mazel, New York

Gull, W.W. (1874) Anorexia nervosa, *Transcripts of the Clinical Society, London, 1*, 22–8

Haley, J. (1959) The family of the schizophrenic: a model system, *Journal of Nervous and Mental Diseases, 129*, 357–74

Halmi, K.A. and Loney, J. (1973) Familial alcoholism in anorexia nervosa, *British Journal of Psychiatry, 123*, 53–4

Halmi, K.A., Strauss, A. and Goldberg, S.C. (1978) An investigation of weights in the parents of anorexia nervosa patients, *Journal of Nervous and Mental Diseases, 166*, 358–61

Kalucy, R.C., Crisp, A.H. and Harding, B. (1977) A study of 56 families with anorexia nervosa, *British Journal of Medical Psychology, 50*, 381–95

Lieberman, S. (1980) *Transgenerational family therapy*, Croom Helm, London

Macleod, S. (1981) *The art of starvation*, Virago, London

Minuchin, S. (1974) *Families and family therapy*, Tavistock Publications, London, pp. 243–4

Minuchin, S., Rosman, B.L. and Baker, L. (1978) *Psychosomatic families: anorexia nervosa in context*, Harvard University Press, Cambridge, MA

Oppenheimer, R., Howells, K., Palmer, R.L. and Chaloner, D.A. (1985) Adverse sexual experience in childhood and clinical eating disorders: a preliminary description, *Journal of Psychiatric Research 19*, 357–61

Palazzoli, M. Selvini- (1974) *Self starvation*, Chaucer, London

Palmer, R.L. (1980) *Anorexia nervosa: a guide for sufferers and their families*, Penguin, London

Palmer, R.L. (1982) Anorexia nervosa. In K. Granville-Grossman (ed.), *Recent Advances in Clinical Psychiatry 4*, Churchill-Livingstone, Edinburgh

Palmer, R.L., Oppenheimer, R. and Marshall, P. (1984) Paper presented at the International Conference on Eating Disorders, Swansea

Szmuckler, G.I., Eisler, I., Russell, G.F.M. and Dare, C. (1985) Anorexia nervosa, parental 'expressed emotion' and dropping out of treatment,

British Journal of Psychiatry, 147, 265–71

Theander, S. (1970) Anorexia nervosa, a psychiatric investigation of 94 female cases, *Acta Psychiatrica Scandinavica (Supplement), 214,* 1–194

Wilkinson, H. (1984) *Puppet on a string,* Hodder and Stoughton, London

Winokur, A., March, V. and Mendels, J. (1980) Primary affective disorder in relatives of patients with anorexia nervosa, *American Journal of Psychiatry, 137,* 695–8

7

Senile Dementia and the Family

Mary L.M. Gilhooly

INTRODUCTION

Every year thousands of people find that they must care for elderly relatives who can no longer remember where they are or what day it is, who have difficulty speaking, and whose forgetfulness leads to the need for help in managing the activities of daily living. For a long time it was believed that this would happen to all people, if they lived long enough. Today, of course, we know that dementia, or, as it is commonly called, 'senility', is caused by disease processes and is not simply an inevitable part of ageing.

This chapter is about coping with senile dementia in the family. It is divided into two parts. In Part I the experiences of the family in caring for a dementing relative will be examined. In Part II a variety of forms of management and intervention with families will be considered. However, the nature of dementia in the elderly, and what is known about its epidemiology, will be briefly outlined first.

The nature of senile dementia

Senile dementia refers to a global and progressive impairment of intellect. There is impairment of memory, especially a failure to register recent events. Emotional changes and personality changes, exaggerated or reversed, commonly accompany senile dementia. In addition to the psychological changes of senile dementia, aphasia is common.

The irreversible dementias of old age are frequently classified into two types. The most common type has been termed 'senile dementia of the Alzheimer's type' (SDAT). Alzheimer's disease was originally described as a presenile dementia (before age 65), but recent evidence has led researchers to question the distinction between Alzheimer's disease and senile dementia. In both pathological changes include the appearance of abnormal structures in the brain such as plaques, neurofibrillary tangles and granulovacuolar structures (Wurtman, 1985). The other main type of dementia is multi-infarct dementia. This type of dementia is caused by small strokes. Multi-infarct dementia is distinguished from SDAT clinically by a characteristic step-wise decline, with gradual deterioration being associated with SDAT.

The epidemiology of the dementias of old age

Because one of the main forms of help offered by professionals to relatives caring for dementing seniors is information, the epidemiology of dementia will be briefly reviewed. The reader should see the referenced papers for more comprehensive accounts.

Prevalence and incidence

Estimates of the prevalence (i.e. all existing cases) of dementia range from around 5 to 15 per cent (Miller, 1977). It is common for a figure of 10 per cent to be cited as the percentage of those over age 65 with dementia. However, this is likely to be an exaggeration, and this figure may well include those suffering from delirium and depression. Mortimer, Schuman and French (1981) note that the median from available surveys is that 4.15 per cent of people over age 65 have definite symptoms of dementia.

There have been few studies of the incidence of dementia (i.e. new cases) in the general population. Akesson (1969) found a 3-year incidence of 0.38 per cent for senile psychosis and 0.52 per cent for arteriosclerotic psychosis. Bergmann, Kay, Foster, McKechnie and Roth (cited by Henderson, 1986) reported an annual incidence rate of 0.8 per cent for senile dementia and 0.7 per cent for arteriosclerotic dementia.

Age

Although the prevalence and incidence of dementia is not known with any precision, there is now abundant evidence that prevalence increases steeply with age. Kay, Bergmann, Foster, McKechnie and Roth (1970) reported prevalence rates of 2.3 per cent in the age group 65–69, rising to 22 per cent in the over-80s. There is also confirmation that the increase in prevalence is due to a rising incidence rate (Akesson, 1969; Hagnell, Lanke, Rorsman, Ohman, and Ojesjo, 1983).

Gender differences in dementia

The evidence to date does not come down clearly on either side of the question of gender or sex differences in the incidence of dementia. Kay (1972) reported identical rates of 'chronic brain syndrome' for men and women, but higher rates of 'senile dementia' for women and higher rates of 'vascular dementia' for men. Broe, Akhtar, Andrews, Caird, Gilmore and McLennan (1976) and Larsson, Sjogren and Jacobsen (1963) found no gender differences for senile dementia. Adelstein, Downham, Stein and Susser (1968) found that women had somewhat higher rates of 'senile psychosis' than men, and Gurland and his colleagues (Gurland, Dean, Cross and Golden, 1980) also found that women had higher prevalence rates of dementia. Although it may still be found to be true that there is a higher incidence of dementia among females than among males, any differences noted so far are usually explained as being due to the more favourable survival rates that women experience in old age.

Family patterns

It is not uncommon for relatives to ask if dementia is inherited. The best answer at the moment is that some forms of dementia may have a genetic factor. There certainly are families in which the incidence of dementia is relatively high. Larsson *et al.* (1963) found a fourfold increase in the probability for first-degree relatives of SDAT patients developing the disease. However, Mortimer *et al.* (1981) have criticised the data collection of this study and, reviewing the literature, suggest that there is evidence of an increased risk among relatives of patients with an onset of Alzheimer's disease before the age of 65, but little risk for relatives of patients with disease of later onset. Evidence that SDAT may be related to Down's syndrome has also led investigators to suspect a genetic factor. Thus, it is probably best to say no more than that the individual may have inherited a tendency to be more vulnerable to the disease, but not that he or she will necessarily develop dementia (Mace and Rabins, 1981).

I. COPING WITH DEMENTIA IN THE FAMILY

The aim of this part of the chapter is to describe and illustrate with case studies some of the problems facing supporters, how supporters cope and the sorts of stresses and strains involved in giving care. The author will draw heavily on her own research on family care of the dementing elderly for this descriptive material.

The author's study consisted of intensive semi-structured interviews with 24 non-resident supporters and 24 co-resident supporters living in Aberdeen in Scotland. The sample was drawn from the records of two day-hospitals, though not all the dementing subjects were attending a day-hospital; the dementing subjects all had a primary diagnosis of senile dementia. Only those with a primary supporter within easy access were included in the study.

The two groups of supporters differed in the following ways: (1) the co-resident supporters were older, (2) the dependants who lived with their supporters were more impaired than those who lived alone, (3) more non-resident supporters had responsibility for another person and were employed, and (4) all the spouse supporters were co-residents. (Details of these differences can be found in Gilhooly, 1984, 1986.)

Even though it was possible to finish the interview in 2–3 hours, depending on family circumstances, most of the interviews took 6–8 hours and were conducted in two or three sessions. The interviews were long because of the supporters' needs to talk to someone about their problems. Few had ever discussed their problems in detail with friends or relatives, and I was the first professional that had ever come along with enough time — and perhaps even enough interest — to talk in depth about their concerns and worries.

Although the qualitative data from these long and detailed interviews will form the basis of this chapter, insights gained by Chris Gilleard and his colleagues in Edinburgh (Gilleard, 1984) and Enid Levin and her colleagues in London (Levin, Sinclair and Gorbach, 1983) will also be utilised. The reader wishing a more detailed literature review of relevant research studies should see Gilleard's book *Living with Dementia*, or some of the articles referenced at the end of the chapter.

The problems of dementia

Clinical descriptions of senile dementia include loss of memory; disorientation for time, place and person; personality changes; and the loosening of inhibitions. But these are not 'problems' for supporters. It is the consequences of these deficits which are problematic for supporters. So, for example, it is not loss of memory that is problematic, it is the inability to remember to put off the gas on the cooker, and the hazards that this in turn creates, that is a problem. Disorientation

141

for time is not a problem; it is getting up in the middle of the night and wandering around the street that is problematic. There is enormous variability in the behaviour that such deficits bring about, and as a consequence what supporters must cope with varies enormously. Add to this the fact that supporters vary widely in what they can tolerate, what they consider to be problematic, and one finds that it becomes difficult to say just what it is about dementia that is so distressing and burdensome for supporters. However, recent research is beginning to show that certain features of dementia do seem to distress most supporters (Gilhooly, 1985; Gilleard, Belford, Gilleard, Whittick and Gledhill, 1984a; Hirschfeld, 1978; Levin et al., 1983). The most disturbing features of dementia appear to be acts of 'commission', rather than acts of 'omission', although there may be overlap between these two categories of behaviour. Since the acts of omission seem to be somewhat less distressing they will be described first.

Acts of omission

(a) Apathy and disinterest. Supporters find it difficult to keep dementing relatives occupied and active. Of course, one can ask why it is that supporters find inactivity distressing. It may be that being 'engaged' or active is a symbol of our humanness, and to see a loved one who is inactive or vegetating but not physically unfit is a reminder that the dementing relative is becoming something else; that his or her 'self' is disintegrating. Keeping a dementing relative active and occupied may also be necessary to prevent other behaviours that are even more distressing from occurring.

The inability to carry on a conversation, or to even show interest in conversations, is also very upsetting for supporters. Lack of mutual conversation is especially difficult for supporters co-residing with the dementing relative if the demands of care-giving have led to social isolation of the primary supporter.

(b) No concern for personal hygiene. Supporters often report that the first sign that something was 'wrong' was when the dementing relative ceased to wash clothes and person. This was then combined with difficulties supporters had in convincing the dementing elder to have a bath, or to agree to let the supporter do the clothes washing.

(c) Not eating properly. Supporters often state that they cannot get their dementing relative to eat anything, or to eat a balanced meal.

Although it could be considered as an act of commission, supporters also worry when dementing elders begin to eat too much of something, usually sweets. One supporter in the author's study found that her mother took to eating constantly; one day she even found her trying to eat paper clips. Supporters often worried that their dementing relatives were leaving food, which either they had prepared or had been left by the meals-on-wheels service, for long periods of time, and therefore risking food poisoning.

Acts of commission

(a) Incontinence. Although incontinence could be seen as an act of omission, it is often the behaviours that surround incontinence that especially disturb supporting relatives. Thus, defaecating in the corner of the living room, hiding wet and soiled underwear, smearing faeces on the wall or self (all behaviours described to me by supporters in my study) are what especially distress supporters. Sometimes these acts of commission are interpreted as deliberate by supporters. Perhaps such interpretations occur because people find it difficult to accept that such behaviours can be a consequence of a disease.

(b) Constant repetition of questions. Because dementing people cannot remember things that have happened in the recent past, they often repeatedly ask the same question. It is rare for supporters to say that they find it easy to cope with constant questioning and their own frustrating attempts to get the answer through to the dementing relative.

(c) Demands for attention. Demands for attention come in two categories — aggressive attention-seeking and an inability to remain alone. Both probably stem from insecurities the dementing person experiences as a result of the inability to remember what the supporter has recently been doing and disorientation for time and place. For example, following the supporter about the house, a common problem for supporters, is probably a consequence of the dementing person's inability to remember where the supporter is and anxieties aroused when the environment seems unfamiliar. This constant demand for attention and the physical presence of the supporter means, of course, that the supporter has little in the way of privacy. One supporter in the author's sample described how she could no longer even shut the door of the toilet because her mother insisted on having her in sight all the time.

(d) Night-time wanderings. In the same way that parents with a new-born baby suffer from the effects of sleep deprivation, supporters co-residing with a dementing person frequently have their sleep disturbed through the night-time wanderings of the dementing person. Months and years on end of disturbed sleep take their toll, and make coping during the day with the demands of care-giving increasingly difficult. Non-resident supporters worry about the dementing person leaving the house and endangering themselves wandering about the streets at night. Non-resident supporters also have their sleep disturbed by middle-of-the-night telephone calls or the arrival at the door of the dementing person. Professionals should not underestimate the devastating effects of these forms of sleep deprivation on supporters.

The daily grind of care-giving

The features described above are those regarded as distressing or problematic by supporters. There are, however, many other impairments with which supporters must cope on a daily basis. Common disabilities include the inability to dress without help, inability to wash without help, falling, inability to eat without help, and inability to get in and out of bed without help. Thus, like many physically disabled persons, the dementing elder comes to need help in most of the activities of daily living. These disabilities, however, combine with acts of commission, making the daily chores of care-giving particularly difficult and frustrating.

To give the reader a feel of what it is like to care for a dementing relative case histories from the author's research will now be described.

Caring for a dementing relative at home — Miss M

Miss M, aged 46, lived with her mother in a high-rise flat. She gave up her job because of a slight health problem and because of the necessity of keeping a constant watch on her mother. Mrs M only went to the day-hospital 2 days a week, Tuesdays and Thursdays. On Tuesdays Miss M went into town to do her shopping and met her sister at lunch time. On Thursdays she went to the hairdresser and again had lunch with her sister.

Miss M's social life was extremely restricted. Besides seeing her sister on Tuesdays and Thursdays, her sister and husband visited, sometimes with their children, on Saturdays.

Mrs M had a living brother and sister, but their own poor health meant that they rarely visited.

There was a neighbour who was quite friendly, but this did not extend to visiting in 'each other's house', and consisted mainly in talking over the balconies.

No practical help was received from this neighbour or from any of the relatives. However, Miss M expressed no resentment at this and her housework seemed to provide something to do. The flat was spotless and a high proportion of time was spent cleaning For example, the windows were cleaned at least once a week.

Miss M busied herself tidying the flat, watching television and, of course, looking after her mother. On the whole Mrs M was not very disabled. She could not, however, cook, clean, prepare a meal or generally participate in housekeeping activities. Mrs M needed some help getting dressed, but did not have to be dressed completely. However, she could not bathe and required extensive help when having a bath. Her hair and general grooming had to be done by her daughter. Mrs M was occasionally incontinent of urine. This problem might have been worse if Miss M did not frequently take her mother to the toilet and supervise.

Helping with dressing, grooming and toileting took up a fair amount of time, but certainly did not fill the day. Miss M could not pursue hobbies or read quietly because her mother followed her around and repeatedly asked questions. Miss M rarely took her mother out. This was for a number of reasons — the embarrassment of unpredictable behaviour, difficulty in getting her ready to go out in bad weather, and the fact that as soon as they got out Mrs M began talking about 'going home'.

Thus, life for Miss M was an endless round of housekeeping chores and television, interspersed by only 2 days of 'relief'. She described how often she wondered if she would make it through the weekend . . . a weekend which started on Thursday at 4 p.m. and ended Tuesday morning at 10. a.m. when the ambulance came again to collect her mother for the day-hospital.

Caring for a non-resident dementing relative — Mrs B

Mrs B was a 55-year-old married daughter. Mrs B's mother was 81 and lived across town in a tenement flat. Mr and Mrs B's son, aged 20, still lived at home. Mrs B worked part-time.

Before Mrs F started attending the day-hospital Mrs B visited her mother every day; the visits were to check on her mother, make sure she was taking her medicines, and generally give her a little company.The schedule at the time of the interview had changed to the following: Sunday, the mother was taken to Mrs B's house for the afternoon and evening. Monday, Mrs B did not visit because Mrs F had a home help; but Mrs B phoned. Tuesday, Mrs B went from work to her mother's house and fixed herself and her mother lunch. She then took her mother out for shopping or a general look around town. Because Mrs F was only mildy confused Mrs B felt it was safe to put her on the bus to go home. Wednesday, Mrs F went to the day-hospital, so her daughter did not visit, but phoned in the evening. Thursday, Mrs B repeated the procedure for Tuesday except she took her mother home and stayed later in the evening, waiting until her husband finished work. Friday, Mrs F went to the day-hospital and Mrs B phoned in the evening. Saturday, Mrs B did not work so collected her mother about noon, took her shopping in the afternoon and then took her home.

It had only been a week from the start of this routine until the interview. Previously, Mrs B had visited her mother every day, and had been visiting every day for 6 months.She said this schedule, with its heavy demands on her time, was a terrible strain and had affected relations within the nuclear family.

As can be seen from these cases it is often not just what one has to do as a supporter for a dementing relative, but what one cannot do, i.e. the effect on one's whole life and relations with other people, that is burdensome and stressful. Supporters vary enormously in how they cope and how they feel about the demands of care-giving. Before describing the methods supporters use to cope, effects on supporters' social and family lives will be described.

Social life

Effects on family life

No matter how well supporters cope with the demands of care-giving, family life will be disrupted or altered in some way. The effects will depend, of course, on the supporter's relation to the dementing elder — spouse, adult child, sibling — and whether or not the supporter is residing in the same home with the dependent person.

If one is caring for a dementing spouse then the first relationship to be affected is that with the spouse. For many supporters, especially females, life may have revolved around the spouse for 40 or 50 years. The cognitive and physical failures accompanying dementia drastically alter that relationship. Supporters frequently feel that their spouse is 'gone' or already dead, and begin grieving before the actual death. Arguments between spouses may begin for the first time. Interestingly, there is evidence suggesting that men cope better and find the change in a spouse easier to adjust to than women. Women appear to be much more emotionally involved in their husbands than men caring for a dementing spouse (Gilhooly, 1984).

Spouse supporters also experience altered relationships with children and sometimes siblings. If adult children aid the spouse supporter, relations within the family may be strengthened. If children do not help, and the spouse supporter feels resentful about lack of help, serious damage to the parent-child relationship can be a consequence. The following story about the effects on relations with adult children was told to the author by one of the respondents in her study, a 76-year-old man who had been looking after his wife for 9 years. This man had five adult children aged 38 to 53. The account below concerned his youngest daughter.

Well really the story was . . . well, they used to ring up once upon a time . . . oh, you could say, every second day, enquiring how their mother was . . . now they haven't been doing that for about a year. . . . Now, how I fell out with the youngest one . . . well, I didn't fall out . . . it was her. . . . She phoned up one day and asked how we were doing . . . 'Oh,' I says, 'I'm not doing too bad but it's a bit of a hermit's life.' . . . Oh, she didn't see it. . . . I was not more of a hermit than she was, and I said, 'What was her complaint? She could get out when the children were at school?' . . . I says, 'What's holding you in?' . . . and eh . . . oh but she thought that [a 13-year-old partially deaf child] was her handicap. . . . I says, 'When [the grandchild] comes up here I find that she helps more than even any of you.' . . . She says, 'Oh, but her temper' . . . I says, 'We know about deaf children and their temper' . . . well, a week elapses and I gets up a piece of paper [in the mail box]. . . . the difficulties mothers have with deaf children, so this was a note in an envelope, nothing who it was from or anything else . . . I said, 'That's a nasty one anyway' . . . now that annoyed me . . . she rang up again in a week's time and she said, 'Do you want assistance or do you want to go out?' . . . 'No,' I says, 'I don't want to go out . . . I've no intention of going out. . . . If I'm needing to go out I'll manage.'

Nearly a year had passed since this incident, and the respondent had not seen this youngest daughter since then. Furthermore, the incident seemed to have affected relations with the other children as well because some had, according to the respondent, taken sides with the daughter, rather than him. This meant that the children were arguing about care-giving and the father's relationships had soured with some of his other children.

This respondent, compared with others in the sample, actually received quite a lot of help and visits from his children (visits at least five times a week and help with shopping, etc.), but felt bitter because he believed that they should be giving more help.

In this case it was hard to know how the children felt about the distribution of care-giving activities, but many of the supporters in the sample who were adult children expressed considerable resentment about lack of help from siblings. What was, however, interesting about relationships between care-givers (and here I am referring mainly to co-resident supporters) and their siblings was that supporters frequently acknowledged that their siblings didn't really know how dependent the dementing parent was, because they had hidden the problems from relatives. Thus, supporters often expressed resentment at lack of help, while at the same time acknowledging that they had never requested help and had kept siblings in the dark about the extent of disability and the stress they were experiencing.

Another aspect of family life that is altered by the demands of caring for a dementing relative in the community is marriage. It should come as no surprise to the reader that marriages are rarely found to improve when one or both partners are supporting a dementing relative. Relationships are no less strained if the dementing relative is not residing with the supporter and supporter's spouse.

In the author's study it was uncommon for adult children to move a dementing relative into their own home. For those supporters and dependants who were co-resident this was a long-standing arrangement (usually due to the shortage of housing after the war and hence the need for a daughter and husband to move in with the daughter's parents). Thus, the dementia had developed long after the couple had accustomed themselves to living with the parent. This may help explain why it is often non-resident supporter spouses who expressed (as reported by the supporter) more resentment about the demands on the supporter's time. It is, of course, likely that husbands who have long lived with a mother-in-law will have grown quite fond of that person, and hence be less likely to complain about time devoted by a wife to care.

One might, of course, argue that when a dementing parent lives with children both children are involved in care-giving. However, this was certainly not true in the author's study. When dementing elders lived with daughters, the daughters' husbands did not share care equally. And when the dementing person was not co-resident, and the dementing person's son was identified as the primary supporter, it was usually found that the son's wife shared the burden of care. Hence, daughters give most of the care with little support from their husbands. This creates considerable role strain for the married supporters, and it was not unusual for married women to say that they would find giving care less stressful if they were not married.

Because prevalence rates for dementia are much higher in older age groups it is unusual for very young children to be residing with co-resident supporters. As a consequence almost nothing is known about the effects of living with a dementing relative on children. The two cases in the author's small sample were, however, reported as having been adversely affected. The effects included behavioural problems at home and at school, and poor academic performance at school. These two children, aged 13 and 14, were also reported as crying more than usual and exhibiting considerable distress about seeing a loved relative deteriorating.

Considerable distress in grandchildren was also reported by non-resident supporters. Many supporters tried to protect their children by reducing visits, and none expected the grandchildren to help in the tasks of care-giving, though some did so.

Effects on relations with friends

Mr W, above, described his life as like a 'hermit'. Although he saw his children regularly, he had almost no contact with neighbours and friends. Partly this was because he and his wife had moved into a smaller council house upon the onset of his wife's dependency and the demands of care made it difficult for Mr W to meet his new neighbours. And, like other supporters in the author's sample, his wife's condition was somewhat of an embarrassment to him so he did not invite people to his house (not that inviting neighbours and friends to one's house is common amongst working-class Aberdonians). Going out to pubs or to friends' houses was impossible because he felt that he could not leave his wife alone.

Not being able to leave the dementing relative alone was a common complaint and frustrating aspect of care-giving for the supporters in the author's sample. Others have also reported that this is a difficulty for supporters (Gilleard, 1984; Hirschfeld, 1978; Levin *et al.*, 1983; Newbigging, 1981). Interestingly the author found that men were more willing than women to leave their dementing spouses alone, locking the door behind them when they left. Most of those supporters who felt that they could not leave their dementing relative alone had become socially isolated.

Non-resident supporters' social lives are also restricted. Visiting dementing relatives — usually every day and sometimes two or three times a day — is time-consuming, leaving little time for social activities. However, in the author's sample many of the non-resident supporters were employed, and their work gave them a social life which was highly valued. Many reported that they could not give support without this social and emotional outlet, and few said that they would be prepared to give up employment to support their dependent relative.

Coping strategies

How supporters of dementing elders cope is virtually unknown. Few studies have attempted to systematically examine coping. Nevertheless, early on in my project I examined the coping strategies of the first 17 respondents in the sample. Use was made of Pearlin and Schooler's (1978) categories of coping, dividing coping firstly into behavioural coping and secondly into psychological coping. Behavioural coping responses include finding out about and making use of health and welfare services and actively organising help from relatives, friends and neighbours. Psychological coping refers to attempts to modify or control the meaning of the stressful experience. There are, of course, numerous ways in which an individual can alter the meaning of a stressful experience.

The categories of psychological coping, taken from Pearlin and Schooler, which were utilised in the analysis were as follows. Each category is illustrated with a case from the author's study.

Making positive comparisons

The hardship is evaluated as being an improvement over the past or as the forerunner of an easier future.

> Mrs T was looking after her 68-year-old husband who was very dependent and incontinent. She was under considerable strain and received little help from her daughters, largely because she refused offers of help. Although very upset, with effects on her physical health as well, Mrs T commented that in one important aspect life had improved for her. Prior to the onset of dementia her husband had been a heavy drinker and frequently came home drunk and

abusive and was sick on the floor. He had since stopped drinking and this was, therefore, an improvement over the past.

Selective ignoring

This involves searching for some positive attribute or circumstance within the stressful experience.

> Mr R was a 35-year-old unmarried son who, along with his father, was caring for his mother. Mr R told the author that there were good things about having to care for a dependent old person, that one learned a lot about ageing and dementia, etc. However, his mother was about to be moved into permanent care and he admitted that had he been interviewed 6 months earlier he might not have been able to say that there had been any 'good' things about giving care.

Re-ordering of life priorities

This involves moving or keeping stressful experiences in the least valued areas of life. The aim is to shrink the significance of problems.

> Mr B was considered by his brothers to be the main supporter to their mother, although he admitted that his wife did as much work as he, perhaps more. He found it very distressing to see his mother deteriorating. However, he stated that his wife and children and his job had to come first, and hence he gave those aspects of his life greater priority.

Converting the hardship into a moral virtue

This method of coping is expressed in sentiments such as 'take the bad with the good', 'try not to worry because time itself solves problems'. This was a common method of coping or thinking about one's position as a supporter. However, it was necessary to divide those who fell into this category into those who felt 'good' about what they were doing and those who did not.

> Mrs G married late in life, and knew that her mother-in-law was dependent when she married. She was quite prepared to take on the role of supporter, and felt that it was only proper and correct that old people should be looked after when they became dependent. However, she received help from her husband and also from her sister-in-law who also lived with the mother. The four

151

people lived in a two-room flat in what can only be described as squalor. However, both Mrs and Mr G were socially active, and though somewhat frustrated about the size of their housing Mrs G expressed little in the way of distress about the demands of care-giving, and believed strongly in 'taking the bad with the good'.

Mrs L had been living with and looking after her mother for 6 years. She was extremely distressed and finding coping very difficult. She could see little that was 'good' in caring for a dementing person, and her only pleasure in giving care seemed to be that she could say to herself that she was doing the 'right' thing. She stated that her mother would not live for ever, and tried telling herself that time would sort out her problems.

These methods of coping psychologically are, of course, only a few of those used by supporters. Understanding the behavioural and psychological strategies used by supporters is, however, important if professionals wish to intervene and help supporters to cope better with the demands of caring for a dementing relative in the community.

The effects of care-giving on psychological well-being

Just how effective the strategies described above, or any others used by supporters, are in helping the supporter is unknown. A very simple analysis of the author's data indicated, as can be seen in Table 7.1, that those using behavioural strategies had higher morale than those using only psychological ones, and those who did not appear to use any of the psychological techniques of cognitively neutralising threats had the lowest morale and were coping least well.

As can also be seen in Table 7.1, those using behavioural coping strategies were predominantly male, and those who were unclassified were female. Gender differences in care-giving were mentioned earlier when describing how men were more willing than women to leave their dementing spouses alone. However, the literature on gender differences in coping and amount of distress experienced when caring for a dementing relative is unclear. Gilleard et al.(1984a) reported higher GHQ scores amongst females than amongst males in three independent samples of supporters of the elderly mentally infirm. Levin et al. (personal communication) also found higher GHQ scores for female supporters than for male supporters, but when the health of female supporters was controlled the gender differences disap-

Table 7.1: Morale score of supporters (by number) making use of behavioural coping responses and the four methods of cognitively neutralising threats described by Pearlin and Schooler (1978). Seven equals high morale and zero low morale

Psychological coping responses	MORALE	Behavioural coping responses	MORALE
1. Making positive comparisons		R2: male	6
R1: female	2	R3: female	6
R13: female	2	R6: male	7
		R8: male	3
2. Selective ignoring		R16: male	4.5
R16: male	4.5		
3. Re-ordering of life priorities		*Unclassified*	
R3: female	6	R5: female	1
R4: female	5	R10: female	1
R6: male	7	R14: female	0
		R12: female	1
4. Converting hardship		R11: female	0
into a moral virtue			
R8: male	3		
R7: female	0		
R9: female	2		

peared. The author (Gilhooly, 1984), using the Kutner Morale Scale, found that males had higher morale than females, but Newbigging (1981), using the same measure of morale, found no gender differences. Finally, Hirschfeld (1978), in a study in San Francisco, found no sex differences in care-givers' management ability, perceived reciprocity of the relationship, level of tension or attitude to institutionalisation. Thus we cannot be certain that care-giving is more stressful for women than for men. Nevertheless, as noted by Judy Zarit (1982), husbands may be able to adopt more effective coping strategies than wives because they can opt out of many needed domestic and personal care chores by utilising traditional sex role models of caring.

Although more research needs to be done to establish the differential effects of caring for a dementing person on women and men, what has, however, been established over the past few years is that caring for a dementing relative is very stressful. Findings are also beginning to accumulate suggesting that caring for the dementing elderly is more stressful than caring for persons with other types of mental disorders, and more stressful than caring for persons who are physically ill.

Gilleard and his colleagues in Edinburgh (1984a) have found

prevalence rates of distress, using the General Health Questionnaire, to be between 57 and 73 per cent. Levin and her colleagues (1983) in London also used the GHQ and found that three-quarters of their sample of supporters of confused old people expressed distress about helping, and a third reported symptoms of acute stress sufficient to suggest a need for psychiatric attention. Greene, Smith, Gardiner and Timbury (1982) in Glasgow, and the Zarits in Los Angeles, have also found that supporters of elderly dementing relatives are under considerable emotional strain (Zarit, 1982; Zarit, Gatz, and Zarit 1981; Zarit, Reever and Bach-Peterson, 1980).

Although there have been no large-scale comparative studies of stress in care-givers, Whittick (1985) found that caring for a dementing relative was more stressful than caring for other types of dependants. Whittick collected data through a postal survey comparing mothers looking after a mentally handicapped child, mothers caring for a mentally handicapped adult, and daughters caring for a dementing parent. Daughters caring for a dementing parent showed higher levels of distress than the mothers caring for a handicapped child or adult. All three groups exhibited greater stress than found in the general population.

Summary

Although little is known about how people cope with caring for a dementing relative, enough research has been conducted to give a picture of what care-giving involves, and the effects of care-giving on care-givers.

The literature is beginning to show that people caring for a dementing relative are under considerable strain, not only in relation to non-care-givers, but in comparison to those caring for other groups of mentally and physically disabled persons. Current knowledge about the aspects of care that supporters find particularly problematic indicates that caring for a dementing person may be quite different from caring for people with other disorders.

There are, however, similarities with other types of care-giving. For example, as with schizophrenia, those caring for dementing people often find it difficult to know whether irritating or distressing behaviours are a consequence of dementia, or deliberately provocative. Supporters of the dementing elderly, like others caring for a mentally ill or handicapped person, frequently hide problems from other relatives and experience anxieties about asking others, including professionals, to share caring.

Finally, when thinking about the 'daily grind' of caring for a dementing relative, and the stresses involved, the reader should keep in mind that those most affected by dementia are women — not only are there more women with dementia than men, but the role of principal care-giver usually falls on women.

II. INTERVENTIONS WITH FAMILIES

Interventions can be placed into three broad categories: (1) counselling; (2) 'practical' or relief services such as home helps, meals on wheels, day care and holiday beds; and (3) institutional care when families can no longer cope with the demands of care-giving. These three types of intervention will be considered now, along with evidence as to whether these services relieve strain or prevent institutionalisation.

Counselling

Counselling with families is of two types: (1) one-to-one counselling with the primary supporter and (2) family meetings. The techniques which can be used are providing information, problem-solving and support. These three techniques can be used in each of the treatment modalities (Zarit and Zarit, 1983).

Information about senile dementia

Supporters are often lacking in knowledge about dementia, frequently not even knowing the diagnosis. Troubling behaviours are interpreted as deliberate provocations by the dependent person, and supporters may believe that the dependent person will get better (Gilhooly, 1982). Such perceptions, of course, make coping difficult. Careful explanation of the disorder, its causes, possibility of cure, role of heredity, etc., is important, but just as important is allowing time and opportunity for questions. Explanation should be supplemented by written material. A recent study by Toner (in review) in Scotland, in which an information booklet was prepared and then evaluated in relationship to supporters' reported stress, indicates that providing written material is very beneficial. Compared to supporters not given a written guide, those given a guide showed significantly greater reductions in GHQ scores over a 5-week period. Follow-up data on a second group of supporters showed a similar reduction in GHQ scores when these supporters were subsequently issued with the information booklet. Toner thought the reductions in distress were more likely to be due to supporters having new information, rather than new skills. Information is often most beneficial because it allows the supporter to re-label troublesome behaviour as illness-related, and hence behaviour which 'can't be helped'.

Problem-solving

Problem-solving involves identifying strategies for modifying the dementing person's behaviour, or the reactions of supporters. Zarit and Zarit (1983) have produced a Memory and Behavior Problems Checklist (see Appendix) which can be useful in identifying specific problem areas which are upsetting for supporters.[1] Record-keeping using checklists such as that devised by Zarit and Zarit often help identify antecedents and consequences of problems which then suggest possible interventions. An example given by Zarit and Zarit is of sleeplessness at night. Record-keeping may reveal that the dementing elder is taking naps during the day, which suggests that keeping the person up and active during the day may reduce sleeplessness at night.

Support

Support from a counsellor can come in three forms. Firstly, there is the support which the counsellor can give by providing an understanding and non-judgemental attitude. Secondly, counsellors can help supporters overcome anxieties about asking other family members, friends or neighbours for help. The research studies by Gilleard, Levin and the author have all revealed that true shared care-giving rarely exists. Often this is because other members of the family gladly hand care to one person. However, it is also true that many supporters, especially women, feel they ought to be able to handle all the caring activities, or that others would not care as well, or that it would be too much of an imposition to ask others for help. The counsellor can help the supporter to identify attitudes such as this which prevent asking for support. Finally, the counsellor can present alternative ways of getting support, such as day-hospital care or holiday breaks.

Family intervention modalities

Three 'treatment' modalities are described by Zarit and Zarit (1983)

— one-to-one counselling, family meetings, and self-help support groups. Little 'formal' one-to-one counselling is offered to relatives of dementing elders in the UK. Family meetings are even less likely to be part of formal counselling, even though they have enormous potential. Self-help support groups have, however, mushroomed all over Britain in recent years.

One-to-one counselling

A private meeting between the primary supporter and the counsellor is most important. Individual sessions help establish the basis for problem-solving and help the counsellor and primary supporter to identify potential help from others. As noted by Zarit and Zarit (1983), the course of this type of counselling will be influenced by the behavioural and cognitive skills of the supporter. Some supporters are effective problem-solvers, but others have difficulty in making changes in how they view a problem.

Family meetings

Zarit and his colleagues at the Andrus Older Adult Center in Los Angeles have found that family meetings bring about impressive changes, with the timely calling of a family meeting frequently making the difference between moderate gain and real success in alleviating the burden on the primary supporter.

The goals of family meetings are (a) to bring the family's level of information up to that of the primary supporter, (b) to identify the supporter's most pressing needs, and (c) to problem-solve with the family to provide more support. The counsellors at the Andrus Older Adult Center have found that family meetings work best if there are two counsellors to chair the meeting. Also, it has been found that counsellors need to be more active initially, especially in answering questions, but that the family members should be encouraged to use their own approaches for giving more support (Zarit and Zarit, 1983).

Self-help support groups

The broad aim of self-help groups for supporters is to relieve supporters of some of the burden they carry in order to fortify them in their care-giving efforts and hence prolong the period of informal care. The participants become acquainted with the dementing process, learn problem-solving and stress management techniques, acquire information on formal supportive services, share common experiences and gain social contacts through group membership (Filinson, 1986).

The impetus for the formation of care-giving support groups

often comes from professionals with a special interest in dementia or the problems of carers. It is often the hope of the professional initiating a support group that the participants will take over the running of the group; the demands of caring for a dementing person mean that this is unlikely.

What happens at a group meeting can vary considerably. There may be professionally facilitated topical presentations, group counselling, instruction in applied skills, or informal, unstructured cathartic discussion sessions (Filinson, 1986). Support groups for care-givers tend to be different from other self-help groups in that their focus is on the entire family unit rather than only individual group participants. Because of this these groups, no matter what the original intention in setting them up, frequently become conduits for emotional outpourings. Zarit (1983) has even suggested that, given the volatile nature of family relationships, candidates for support groups should be screened. Also, because of the sensitive nature of the emotional expressions in such groups, professionals involved should ensure that they have the skills needed to handle the emotions aroused in the group, and to ensure that group norms and processes do not become destructive.

Supporting the supporters with services

For some time it was assumed that care for dementing old people 'broke down', and supporters then requested or demanded institutional care. Furthermore, it was assumed that, if some of the problems of giving care in the community could be alleviated by providing services, supporters would continue to give care. Research evidence to date, however, calls into question such assumptions.

To understand why relatives decide to cease giving support one needs to understand what causes relatives to give care in the first place. An important research question is whether accurate predictions can be made about the duration of care-giving from knowledge of supporters' attitudes to continued care-giving.

As with other aspects of family care of the dementing elderly, very little research has been done on attitudes to care-giving. Why someone gives care to a dementing relative depends, of course, on the blood or role relationship with that person. Spouses in the author's sample often repeated part of their marriage vows, saying that they had promised to love and honour in sickness and in health. Spouses have also been found to be less willing than children or siblings to consider institutional care (Gilhooly, 1986). The adult children in the author's sample gave care out of love, moral obligation, a feeling that they were returning the care given to them when they were children, and, importantly, because they felt that the alternatives to their giving care could not be considered. Partly this was due to the belief that they could give the kindest and best care, and partly because the types of institutional care which were available were too ghastly to contemplate. Many supporters referred to the local psychiatric hospital as the 'asylum', and expressed quite negative views about the hospital. Thus, 'stigma' often prevented supporters giving up the role of supporter, rather than the desire to give care motivating them to continue.

The relationship between the supporter and dependent person — blood/role and quality of the relationship — are, of course, factors which cannot be manipulated by professionals. But what of the role of services such as day-hospital care, home help, and meals-on-wheels in helping supporters to cope? And do services sufficiently reduce stress to delay or prevent institutionalisation?

Here the literature is somewhat conflicting. Taking stress first we find that Levin and her colleagues (1983, 1985) in London found that day care, relief admissions and home helps reduced the build-up of strain in supporters as measured by the GHQ. The author, however, found that, although frequency of home helps and visits from a community psychiatric nurse were associated with morale, frequency of attendance at a day-hospital and meals-on-wheels were not (Gilhooly, 1984). Furthermore, Gilleard and his colleagues in Edinburgh (1984b), Whittick (1985) in Scotland, and Zarit (1982) in Los Angeles found that formal service provision was not associated with reduced burden or improved psychological well-being.

A rather similar picture emerges when one looks at the role of services in preventing or delaying institutionalisation of the dementing person. Levin and her colleagues in London found that the home help service could in certain circumstances postpone or prevent admission to an institution. However, Gilleard (1985) found that the more community and health services were received, the more likely psychogeriatric day-hospital patients were to be institutionalised. Studies have also found that provision of services is not related to attitude to continued care-giving (Gilhooly, 1986; Whittick, 1985; Zarit, 1982). Such findings are relevant because attitude to continued care-giving has been found to be predictive of outcome (Gilleard, 1984; Levin et al., 1983).

Taken as a whole these studies suggest that formal services as currently provided do not prevent institutionalisation; nor do they do a lot to reduce burden or distress. This may be because not enough is provided in the way of services, or because the types of services offered are inappropriate.

It is certainly the case that service provision in Scotland for the dementing elderly and their supporters is low and uniform. For example, in the author's sample most of those dementing elders attending a day-hospital only received 2 days per week of day-hospital care. With such uniformity of service provision, i.e. lack of variation in the independent variable, one is unlikely to find significant correlations with dependent variables such as measures of burden or attitude to continued care-giving. Thus, the lack of a statistical association between service provision and distress or outcome may be due to the nature of statistics, rather than service provision having no impact.

A less optimistic view is that the services currently provided do not meet the needs of those caring for dementing people in the community. If we go back and look at the types of problems which distress supporters most, we see that they are things that require intervention in the dementing person's behaviour, e.g. incontinence. Intervening in a relative's behaviour is likely to be very much more stressful than providing services such as cooking meals. Yet, as noted by Gilleard (1984), what we currently provide is services that supplement the disabilities of the dementing person, rather than supervisory services. If services are to reduce the burden on supporters, and ultimately prevent institutionalisation, then we need to think more imaginatively about the types of services we provide.

Institutional care

Zarit and Zarit (1983) note that in the United States the prevailing approach to treatment of dementia patients is custodial, with physicians and other professionals advising supporters to place their dementing relatives in nursing homes. Because there are few nursing homes in Britain, there are long waiting lists for beds in psychiatric and geriatric hospitals. Old people's homes are reluctant to admit mentally impaired persons. Thus, in Britain there are few alternatives to home care. Nevertheless many dementing people have no relatives, for many supporters the strain of giving care will be so great that institutional care will become necessary to preserve the well-being of the supporter, and there will always be some people who are unwilling to give care to a dementing relative.

Relocation from the community to an institution is known to be a traumatic, if not catastrophic, event for dementing people (Borup, Gallego and Hefferman, 1979, 1980). What is less often appreciated is how traumatic relocation is for relatives. Although there is evidence that institutionalisation relieves the strain of care-giving (Levin *et al.*, 1983, 1985), visiting an institutionalised relative can be very upsetting for supporters. As supporters have an important role to play after institutionalisation takes place, it is worthwhile examining some of the things that upset supporters when they visit their dementing relatives in an institution. The information presented comes from discussions by the author with people who have given up the care-giving role, usually reluctantly.

Upsetting features of institutional care

It often comes as a great shock for supporters to see their dementing relative surrounded by other dementing people. Though staff may think that all the patients are about equally disabled, supporters tend to report that their relative is somehow different. That is, supporters frequently report either that their dementing relative is less mentally impaired than the other patients, or that they had not realised until their first visit that their relative was so seriously mentally impaired. No matter how these perceptions are reported, what is clear is that supporters perceive their own relative as a 'person' with problems related to mental state, with the other residents being perceived of as patients. Supporters have even reported to me that they didn't want their relatives to be with other dementing people.

Besides feeling upset at the sight of one's own relative, and being upset by the sight of numbers of dementing people who may be behaving strangely, supporters frequently report being upset because there is no place where they can talk privately with the person they are visiting. It will be some time before patients in psychiatric hospitals in the UK have private or even double-bedded rooms, but it does not seem unreasonable that a room be set aside for private visiting near long-stay wards.

Bereavement counselling

Bereavement counselling is usually offered after a death. However, relatives of institutionalised dementing people often experience the relocation of the dependant as a bereavement. The supporter may experience many or all of the phases or stages of bereavement described by Parkes (1972) and others. The professional's concern with the family should not end upon the institutionalisation of the

161

dementing person. The following part of an interview with a woman whose husband had been admitted to a long-stay ward in a psychiatric hospital indicates how supporters feel.

MG — How do you feel now? Do you feel any happier now?

R — No. [said very softly]

MG — How exactly do you feel? I mean, you don't have the stress and strain of caring for your husband.

R — No, uhuh. Ah wis oot seein' him on Sunday an' ah wis really broken haerted. [respondent begins to cry]

MG — I don't want to upset you.
 [pause]

MG — Have you felt lonely since your husband left?

R — Well . . . depressed.

MG — Now, since your husband went out to the hospital, has anyone from the services come to see you?

R — No.

MG — Have you had any help?

R — No, no, nup, nup.

MG — When your husband was here, of course, in a sense you were like a nurse, it was like a job being a nurse . . .

R — Aye, yes you'd ties . . .

MG — Do you feel now that you're not doing this nursing that you haven't a purpose or role in life?

R — (short pause) No, ah hinna a role in life now, no. Ah ging tae me bed in the aefterneens, my bed in the aefterneens, nowaday, yes.

MG — Is that because you're tired?

R — Nae tired, really to shove in time. . . .

As can be seen, this supporter was very upset by the relocation of her husband. She had been taking tranquillisers when caring for her husband and was still taking them. She cried during most of the interview but said that it felt good to be able to talk about her husband. I was the only 'professional' to have visited since the admission of her husband to hospital, and the main aim of my visit was to collect data for a research project.

Most supporters will, of course, cope with their feelings on their own, but they need to know that there is someone willing to listen and help, should they need it.

Summary

A variety of ways in which professionals can help those giving care in the community to dementing relatives were outlined in this section of the chapter. Some of these methods of helping (e.g. counselling via family meetings, self-help support groups) have yet to be systematically evaluated, so we do not know whether or not they relieve burden or prevent institutionalisation. Nevertheless, research is beginning to show that traditional ways of giving support may not be as effective as expected. Moreover, because many relatives cannot sustain care in the community, ways of involving supporters in institutional care should also be introduced. Lastly, the trauma that supporters experience when their dementing relative is admitted to institutional care should be acknowledged through supportive services.

CONCLUSION

It would have been nice to have been able to spend time in this chapter outlining what can be done to help dementing people cope with their illness. Unfortunately there is no cure, and although drugs may control certain symptoms, in many cases symptoms are exacerbated by drugs. The evidence on therapies like Reality Orientation is not encouraging, although this may have as much to do with the way it has been practised as its real effectiveness (Hanley, 1984). Nevertheless practising Reality Orientation may be beneficial for some relatives; at least they feel they are doing something to help the dementing person.

Although this may sound like bad news for professionals dealing with dementing seniors, the good news is that professionals can do a lot to help carers. A cautionary note should, however, be added. The forms of intervention outlined in this chapter are unlikely to help those who do not want to give care. Moreover, the numbers of relatives who want to care for their dementing relatives in the community may be smaller than government officials and administrators might wish (West, Illsley and Kelman, 1984). Given that institutional care will be the first choice of care for many relatives, professionals need to think imaginatively of ways to get relatives involved in care after institutionalisation, plus ways of improving institutional care for dementing people.

NOTE

1. Chris Gilleard has also developed a Problem Check List, which assesses frequencies of problems and the amount of distress the problems cause for the care-giver. Gilleard's Problem Check List has been used only for research purposes and not for counselling.

REFERENCES

Adelstein, A.A., Downham, D.Y., Stein, Z. and Susser, M.W. (1968) The epidemiology of mental illness in an English city, *Journal of Social Psychiatry, 3*, 47–59

Akesson, H.O. (1969) A population study of senile and arteriosclerotic psychosis, *Human Heredity, 19*, 546–66

Borup, J.H., Gallego, D. and Hefferman, P. (1979) Relocation and its effects on mortality, *Gerontologist, 19*, 135–40

Borup, J.H., Gallego, D. and Hefferman, P. (1980) Relocation: its effects on health functioning and mortality, *Gerontologist, 20*, 468–79

Broe, G.A., Akhtar, A.J., Andrews, G.R., Caird, F.I., Gilmore, A.J.J. and McLennan, W.J. (1976) Neurological disorders in the elderly at home, *Journal of Neurology, Neurosurgery and Psychiatry, 39*, 362–6

Filinson, R. (1986) Self-help and family support groups. In I. Hanley and M.L.M. Gilhooly (eds), *Psychological therapies for the elderly*, Croom Helm, Beckenham; New York University Press, New York, pp. 101–23

Gilhooly, M.L.M. (1982) Social aspects of senile dementia. In R. Taylor and A. Guilmore (eds), *Current trends in British gerontology: Proceedings of the 1980 Conference of the British Society of Gerontology*, Gower Press, Aldershot, pp. 61–76

Gilhooly, M.L.M. (1984) The impact of care-giving on care-givers: factors associated with the psychological well-being of people supporting a dementing relative in the community, *British Journal of Medical Psychology, 57*, 35–44

Gilhooly, M.L.M. (1985) Community care of the dementing elderly: is it really feasible? Paper presented to the annual conference of the Association of Psychiatric Nurses, Aberdeen, 18 October

Gilhooly, M.L.M. (1986) Senile dementia: factors associated with caregivers' preference for institutional care, *British Journal of Medical Psychology, 59*, 165–71

Gilleard, C.J. (1984) *Living with dementia: community care of the elderly mentally infirm*, Croom Helm, London; Charles Press, Philadelphia

Gilleard, C.J. (1985) Predicting the outcome of psychogeriatric day care, *Gerontologist, 25*, 280–5

Gilleard, C.J., Belford, H., Gilleard, E., Whittick, J.E. and Gledhill, K. (1984a) Emotional distress amongst supporters of the elderly mentally infirm, *British Journal of Psychiatry, 145*, 172–7

Gilleard, C.J., Gilleard, E., Gledhill, K. and Whittick, J. (1984b) Caring for the elderly mentally infirm at home: a survey of the supporters, *Journal of Epidemiology and Community Health, 38*, 319–25

Greene, J.G., Smith, R., Gardiner, M. and Timbury, G.C. (1982) Measuring behavioural disturbance of elderly demented patients in the community and its effects on relatives: a factor analytic study, *Age and Ageing, 11*, 121–6

Gurland, B.J., Dean, L., Cross, P. and Golden, R. (1980) The epidemiology of depression and dementia in the elderly: the use of multiple indicators of these conditions. In J.O. Cole and J.E. Barrett (eds), *Psychopathology in the aged*, Raven Press, New York,

Hagnell, O., Lanke, J., Rorsman, B., Ohman, R. and Ojesjo, L. (1983) Current trends in the incidence of senile and multi-infarct dementia: a prospective study of a total population followed over 25 years: the Lundby Study, *Archives of Psychiatry and Neurological Science, 233*, 423–38

Hanley, I. (1984) Theoretical and practical considerations in reality orientation therapy with the elderly. In I. Hanley and J. Hodge (eds), *Psychological approaches to the care of the elderly*, Croom Helm, London; Methuen, New York, pp. 164–91

Henderson, A.S. (1986) The epidemiology of Alzheimer's disease *British Medical Bulletin, 42*, 3–10

Hirschfeld, M.J. (1978) Families living with senile brain disease. Dissertation submitted in partial satisfaction of the requirements for the degree of Doctor of Nursing Science, University of California, San Francisco

Kay, D.W.K. (1972) Epidemiological aspects of organic brain disease in the aged. In C.M. Gates (ed), *Aging and the brain*, Plenum Press, London

Kay. D.W.K., Bergmann, K., Foster, E.M., McKechnie, A.A. and Roth, M. (1970) Mental illness, hospital usage in the elderly: a random sample followed up, *Comprehensive Psychiatry, 11*, 26–35

Larsson, T., Sjogren, T. and Jacobsen, G. (1963) Senile dementia: a clinical, socio-medical and genetic study, *Acta Psychiatrica Scandinavica, Suppl.*, *167*, 1–259

Levin, E., Sinclair, I. and Gorbach, P. (1983) The supporters of confused elderly persons at home: Extract from the Main Report. National Institute for Social Work Research Unit, London

Levin, E., Sinclair, I. and Gorbach, P. (1985) The effectiveness of the home help services with confused old people and their families, *Research, Policy and Planning, 3*, 1–7

Mace, N. and Rabins, P. (1981) *The 36-hour day*, Johns Hopkins University Press, Baltimore

Miller, E. (1977) *Abnormal ageing: the psychology of senile and presenile dementia*, John Wiley, London

Mortimer, J.A., Schuman, L.M. and French, L.R. (1981) Epidemiology of dementing illness. In J.A. Mortimer and L.M. Schuman (eds), *The epidemiology of dementia*, Oxford University Press, Oxford, pp. 3–23

Newbigging, K. (1981) 'A ripe old age?': an investigation of relatives of elderly dependants with dementia. Thesis submitted in part fulfilment of the requirements for the British Psychological Society Diploma in Clinical Psychology

Parkes, C.M. (1972) *Bereavement: studies of grief in adult life*, Penguin, London

Pearlin, L.I. and Schooler, C. (1978) The structure of coping, *Journal of Health and Social Behavior, 19,* 2–21

Toner, H. (in review) Evaluation of the effectiveness of a written guide for carers of dementia sufferers

West, P., Illsley, R. and Kelman, H. (1984) Public preferences for the care of dependency groups, *Social Science and Medicine, 18,* 287–95

Whittick, J.E. (1985) Attitudes to caregiving. Dissertation submitted to the University of Edinburgh in partial fulfilment of an M.Phil.

Wurtman, R.J. (1985) Alzheimer's disease, *Scientific American, 252,* 62–74

Zarit, J.M. (1982) Predictors of burden and distress for caregivers of senile dementia patients. Unpublished doctoral dissertation, University of Southern California

Zarit, S.H. (1983) Interventions with families of impaired elderly. Paper presented at the 36th Annual Scientific Meeting of the Gerontological Society of America, San Francisco

Zarit, S.H. and Zarit, J.M. (1983) Cognitive impairment of older persons: etiology, evaluation and intervention. In P.M. Lewinsohn and L. Teri (eds), *Coping and adaptation in the elderly,* Pergamon Press, New York

Zarit, J.M., Gatz, M. and Zarit, S.H. (1981) Family relationship and burden in long-term care. Paper presented at the 34th Annual Scientific Meeting of the Gerontological Society of America, Toronto, Canada, November

Zarit, S.H., Reever, K.E. and Bach-Peterson, J. (1980) Relatives of the impaired elderly: correlates of feelings of burden, *Gerontologist, 20,* 649–55

APPENDIX: MEMORY AND BEHAVIOUR PROBLEMS CHECKLIST

Instructions to interviewer

This checklist is administered in two parts. In Part A the frequency with which problems occur is determined. In Part B it is determined to what degree the behaviour upsets the care-giver. When you find out that a problem occurs, then ask if it is upsetting.

Instructions to care-giver

'I am going to read you a list of common problems. Tell me if any of these problems have occurred during the past week. If so, how often have they occurred? If not, has this problem ever occurred?' For Part B — 'How much does this problem bother or upset you?'

Frequency ratings	Reaction ratings: How much does this bother or upset you when it happens?
0 = never occurred	0 = not at all
1 = has occurred but not in past week	1 = a little
2 = has occurred one or two times in past week	2 = moderately
3 = has occurred three to six times in past week	3 = very much
4 = occurs daily or more often	4 = extremely
7 = would occur, if not supervised by care-giver (e.g. wandering except door is locked)	
8 = patient never performed this activity	

167

Behaviours

1. Wandering or getting lost
2. Asking repetitive questions
3. Hiding things (money, jewellery, etc.)
4. Being suspicious or accusative
5. Losing or misplacing things
6. Not recognising familiar people
7. Forgetting what day it is
8. Not completing tasks
9. Destroying property
10. Doing things that embarrass you
11. Waking you up at night
12. Being constantly restless
13. Being constantly talkative
14. Engaging in behaviour that is potentially dangerous to others or self (interviewer's judgement for whether behaviour is dangerous or merely troublesome)
15. Reliving situations from the past
16. Seeing or hearing things that are not there (hallucinations or illusions)
17. Unable to dress self (partly or totally)
18. Unable to feed self
19. Unable to bathe or shower by self
20. Unable to put on make-up or shave by self
21. Incontinent of bowel or bladder
22. Unable to prepare meals
23. Unable to use phone
24. Unable to handle money
25. Unable to clean the house
26. Unable to shop
27. Unable to do other simple tasks — specify (e.g. put groceries away, simple repairs)
28. Unable to stay alone by self
29. Other (specify)

8

Violence Towards Wives

R. Emerson Dobash and Russell P. Dobash

In this chapter we will consider the extent of wife abuse, provide a description of the violent event in terms of the attack, injuries and immediate responses, analyse the nature of help-seeking behaviour of women who are abused and consider the response of agencies to the victims, abusers and the problem in general. This approach provides a wider interpretation of a problem that is too often viewed only in terms of attributes of the individuals and/or families involved, without due consideration of the social and cultural contexts in which it occurs and through which it can be best understood.

THE EXTENT OF VIOLENCE AGAINST WIVES: HOMICIDES AND ASSAULTS

Studies of the incidence of assaults and homicides in Britain, North America and on the European continent reveal several basic patterns: males are far more likely to be violent than females; when women are involved in violent incidents it is usually as victims and not as perpetrators; when males are victims of violence it is usually outside the family setting and at the hands of an unrelated male; and finally, when females are victims of violence it usually occurs inside the family setting and is at the hands of a male relative, usually her husband or cohabitant (Dobash and Dobash, 1979). While the majority of murders are committed by an acquaintance or relative of the victim, women are more likely to be killed by their spouse while men are more likely to be killed by someone outside the family. Studies of murder in England and Wales show that, when women are killed, it is usually by their husband or cohabitant, and the same pattern has been found in many American studies (Gibson and Klein, 1969;

Gibson, 1975). Wolfgang's (1958) classic study of violent crime in Philadelphia, and Voss and Hepburn's (1968) research in Chicago, both revealed that female victims of homicide were usually married to their assailants.

Analysis of police records and self-report studies of victims in the United States and Britain reveals that wife-beating is widespread and represents a considerable proportion of all violent offences dealt with by the police and courts (Gaguin, 1978; Worrall and Pease, 1986). For example, in the 1950s and early 1960s 'domestic disputes' accounted for 30 per cent of all violent offences dealt with by the London police, and 90 per cent of those were wife assaults (McClintock, 1963). Our own research in Scotland, which involved an analysis of court and police records for one year in Edinburgh and a major district in Glasgow, showed that the majority of the 33,724 cases analysed involved traffic offences (41 per cent) and non-violent breaches of the peace, theft and other miscellaneous offences (48 per cent), with less than 10 per cent involving any type of violence. Of the 3020 violent cases, two categories occurred more frequently than all others: violence between unrelated, though often acquainted, males (38.7 per cent, 1169 cases) and wife assaults (25.1 per cent, 759 cases). There were only 12 assaults on husbands by their wives (0.4 per cent). The majority of all violent offenders in domestic and non-domestic settings were males (91.4 per cent), yet victims were almost equally distributed between males (55.3 per cent) and females (44.6 per cent). This over-representation of women as victims in the crime statistics is even more significant when we examine the gender of offender and victim in cases of violence in the home. While 97.4 per cent of the offending family members were male, 94.4 per cent of the victims were females (Dobash and Dobash, 1977, 1978).

Police records provide only a partial indication of how widespread wife-beating actually is, since they cannot include cases not reported to them and do not include those in which they failed to bring a charge (Wasoff, 1982). Violence against wives continues to be an unshareable and hidden problem, and some women endure violence for years without telling anyone or before seeking assistance. Of course this means that police records and self-report studies give a much lower indication of the violence than actually occurs: of the women we interviewed, only two out of every 98 assaults they received throughout their married lives were reported to the police. Despite this vast under-reporting and under-recording, these sources still show that wife abuse is a serious and significant problem, and that women are far more likely to be killed or assaulted by their spouse than by anyone else.

This pattern indicates the importance of seeing much of the violence used against women as related to their social position as wives.

THE CONTEXT-SPECIFIC APPROACH

Providing an explanation of any social problem is a necessary step in working toward a solution, and yet much more is required in the way of analysis of this problem than social scientists have usually provided. The task of explanation requires that we analyse the accounts of those who have experienced the problem, and seek to discover the more general patterns revealed in their collective experiences. Individual experiences are not, however, sufficient to provide an adequate explanation; they must be in turn placed in the overall context of the society in which they occur. This wider analysis must include a careful consideration of the historical legacy of the problem, as well as contemporary social arrangements and cultural beliefs concerning the positions of men and women. The context-specific approach we adopted in our research begins by focusing on the problem of wife-beating and places this in the numerous contexts in which it occurs (see Dobash and Dobash, 1979, 1983 for a fuller discussion). In ever-widening circles we examine the violent event, individuals and their relationships, social beliefs and practices, institutional policy and practice, and finally the historical legacy of wife-beating.

In order to do this we analysed police and court records for a one-year period, conducted in-depth interviews with 109 battered women, examined current social and legal policies and practices and investigated the historical legacy of wife-beating. The context-specific approach to the problem of wife-beating locates it firmly within the diverse contexts in which it occurs — personal, interactional, cultural, institutional and historical. Such a methodology contrasts sharply with the more narrow focus on individual deviance or pathology.

The problem of wife-beating is not primarily the result of deviant subcultures, pathological personalities of men or of so-called violence-prone or masochistic women, but is firmly embedded in widely accepted and cherished ideals and patterns of behaviour, such as male aggressiveness and authority and female dependence and subordination. As such we do not need to seek the answer to wife-beating in analyses that merely attempt to parcel out various deviant factors associated with those couples experiencing the problem. Men who beat their wives are, in a most obvious and brutal fashion, living up to many values and ideals still cherished in our society.

171

An important aspect of our method was a detailed exploration of specific violent events. Researchers often concentrate only on the characteristics of the individuals involved in violence, or the meanings attached to human actions, and fail to consider the concrete circumstances of daily life. By contrast we investigated the complexity of violent events and their aftermath as a means of understanding the reality of women's lives. We asked them about three specific violent incidents, the first, the worst and the last they experienced before going to a refuge. Some of the areas covered included the circumstances preceding the violence, the physical nature of the attack, its location, the extent and severity of injuries, and men's and women's reactions during and immediately following the attack. We also asked about the features of a usual, or typical, violent event. This enabled us to develop thorough descriptions of violent events, to distil their most significant features and to assess the changes in violence over time. In the following section we will consider the usual nature of this violence.

THE NATURE OF VIOLENT EVENTS

Physical force

The types of physical force used during a violent episode are quite varied and include such things as slapping, pushing and shoving, punching, kicking, kneeing, butting, striking with or throwing household objects, the use of weapons and attempts to smother or strangle. We found that the most common form of physical force was repeated punching to the face and/or body, and the second most common type involved kicking, kneeing and butting (Dobash and Dobash, 1984). Almost half of the women we interviewed said that punching was a major feature of the attacks they experienced. Kicking, butting or kneeing occurred less frequently, with 28 per cent of the women reporting it as a typical element of assaults. Another very common form of violence is pushing, pulling or shoving, and, while one might think this is a rather innocuous form of violence, its severity depends on many factors such as where the man grabs the woman when pulling and shoving her, and whether the object is soft such as a sofa or bed, or hard such as a wall or stairs.

We also discovered numerous incidents involving strangulation or suffocation, as well as beatings with objects such as lamps or tables, and a whole host of other forms of violence including burning, biting, urinating and standing or jumping on women, threatening them with weapons and rape.

> Oh he's tried to strangle me more than once. He'd put his hands around my throat and he'd fire certain questions. If you kind of wanted to save your life, you had to give him the answers that he required. Then he might let go.

In general we found, as have other researchers (Binney, Harkell and Nixon, 1981; Evason, 1982), that a violent attack usually consisted of several different kinds of physical violence used repeatedly.

Injuries

A wide variety of injuries were sustained from such acts of violence, including bruises, cuts, broken bones and teeth, and miscarriages, but the most common form of injury was multiple bruising. Bruising accounted for nearly three-quarters of the injuries in the first, worst and last assaults, and it was often quite massive, covering a sizeable area of the face and/or body. The second most common injury was cuts, but the list of injuries seems endless and as varied as the attacks.

> Oh, my mouth was bleeding and I'd lost a tooth. In fact I've still got one of the kick marks up here [on the face]. You couldn't count the number of black eyes. See it's a long time, eighteen years.

> He pulled all my hair out here, and my legs were all bruised.

Most women experienced a variety of injuries during a single violent episode, and many required medical treatment. Yet in numerous instances they did not receive this necessary attention, either because they were physically prevented from leaving the house or threatened with reprisals if they did. Some women had to strike a bargain that if allowed to receive treatment they would not reveal the source of injuries.

Women's responses

The invisible injuries of fear, tension and depression also took a high toll and affected almost every woman. This included the fear during an assault, tension and apprehension between the attacks, and the more general sense of anxiety and depression.

> I often feel like jumping through the window just to put an end to it. And often I see cars and buses and I'll say, now if I just walk in front of them, if they're going hard enough, they'd just kill me quick, and that would be it. You often wonder what your life is . . . if this is all your life's going to be.

> I'm terrified of him. I've got more guts now than I've ever had, but I'm still terrified of him. If I'd see him now I'd run a mile, I would really run a mile.

Such emotions are far more likely after being subjected to violence for a prolonged period.

In the beginning, when the violence is less frequent and severe, women have considerable hope for reformation, the cessation of violence and a successful marriage. Rarely is the first assault as severe as subsequent ones. It is usually more shocking to the woman, and sometimes the man, but it is more readily forgiven and forgotten. There is no reason to see this as the beginning of a pattern and it is usually treated as an 'isolated' event. At this stage it is precisely that. After the first violent event, men are contrite and express remorse. This, along with more general ideals about the importance of marriage, leads women to forgive them and to try to work on changing the marriage so that violence might be eliminated. Over time, the violence increases in frequency and severity (an average of twice a week). Women eventually begin to redefine the man's attacks as persistent, their marriages as violent and themselves as battered wives. They lose hope, feel trapped and begin, usually with reluctance, to seek assistance from outsiders. But what factors lead to these violent events?

CIRCUMSTANCES LEADING TO VIOLENCE

Violent episodes do not have a precise beginning or ending, but are a continuous process with the ending of one episode forming the beginning of the next, particularly as long-standing disagreements and the injustice of violent attacks shape the bridges between them. As such it is impossible to encapsulate a violent episode and set it apart from the patterns of authority, domestic life and sources of disagreement that constitute integral aspects of each event and of the contentious issues that link one event to the next. Two general sources of argument lead to over half of all of the violent incidents in our study — the husband's possessiveness or sexual jealousy, and his expectations concerning the woman's domestic work.

Domestic work

Arguments about domestic work were often about the timing of meals and/or the type of food served, with men expecting meals to be served immediately upon their arrival at any hour of the day or night. Any lack of speed or reluctance to comply might be seen both as a failure of the wifely duty to serve him and a challenge to his authority over her.

The beliefs in a husband's authority and a wife's obligation to serve are evident throughout British society and not just among men who physically attack their wives. The difference is that some men are prepared to use violence to enforce them. The following illustrates how stringently this can be held:

It was a Sunday and I went up to my mother's. I came in and he was in a bad mood because I'd went to my mother's and he said he was hungry. I'd made him mince and potatoes for his dinner but he wouldn't [heat it]. He'll make nothing for himself, and he started moaning because I wasn't there to make it and he just knocked hell out of me.

Another woman said that the first time she was ever subjected to physical abuse was because her husband didn't like what she served him.

No, no argument. It wasn't what he wanted for his tea so he threw it at me. Well, I had the dinner all down my front, and I got a bruised chest. I was speechless. I just stood and looked at him. I burst into tears and went away out. I was very upset about it. I mean, I had never seen anything like this happening. I'd never experienced violence in a home.

Violent incidents occurred because of meals that were a few minutes late, or food deemed unacceptable, such as a cheese sandwich rather than a ham sandwich. Other attacks began because of the woman's

175

reluctance to get out of bed and cook a meal late at night, or because a meal had become dry sitting in the oven for hours waiting upon the man's late arrival, or simply because a particular meal or the way it was served did not please him.

There are many other aspects of domestic work where the man feels that he has the right to dictate almost any kind of demand for service no matter how unrealistic or unjust, and to punish or correct failures by various means, including the use of violence. Domestic work was the source of conflict in 16 per cent of the typical attacks. While the specific issues may seem trivial, a greasy egg or a cheese sandwich, it is the husband's authority and his conceptions of the woman's duty to serve him that are the factors leading to violence. His sense of rightful authority provides the justification for his actions, and is also the means by which he transfers the blame for his own actions to the woman.

Possessiveness

The other major source of conflict leading to assaults is the man's possessiveness. Almost half (45 per cent) of the typical assaults centred on objections representing the husband's possessiveness. For many women, conducting their daily lives of shopping, engaging in discussions with a repair man, or even giving directions to a male passer-by was nearly impossible without their husbands becoming jealous. For most women it was impossible to convince their husbands that there was no cause for jealousy.

> Well, I tried to get through to him that I never had a relationship with another man. But I mean, I couldn't get through to him at all. It was like trying to hammer a nail into that wall, you can't do it unless you put a plug in it. He just would not have it, he just kept saying the same old things, I'd been out with every Tom, Dick and Harry. I says, 'I've been honest with you. I've never had intercourse with another man in all the years, neither before we got married nor after.' Well, one day he turned around and said, 'Well in that case you're a nun and I can't live with a nun.'

Despite changes in the position of women in our society, marriage is still not an egalitarian relationship, the patriarchy is not dead and a double standard still exists. Although both husbands and wives may feel possessive about their spouse, it is men who have learned to have the greatest expectations and are most sensitive to behaviour perceived as a deviation or an affront. For men, the possession of their wives is not only personally desirable, but also an outward indication that they are truly men, that is, in control of their wives. This explains a great deal about the inordinate demands many men make on their wives.

Money

The third most common source of conflict leading to an assault was money; 17 per cent of typical attacks involved such a focus (Pahl, 1983). There was considerable variation in the types of problems associated with money, but most were basically about how much was available for housekeeping and how much the men used on their own pursuits and recreation. Women often had to extricate the house-keeping in the first place, and then negotiate when he wanted to take it back for his own use. Many altercations occurred because women were expected to manage the household and provide large, hearty meals on impossibly small sums of money while husbands spent the rest on their own clothing and leisure pursuits.

It was in connection with money, and with the amount of time the husband spends away from home, that the issue of drinking was likely to become a topic of contention. For a few couples the husband's drinking *per se* was a source of conflict leading to an assault, but in general this was far less usual than popular mythology would have us believe. In our police study we found a quarter of the men processed for attacks on wives were described as drunk, and this corresponds closely with the findings in American studies. It is very likely that the higher rate in police cases reflects the filtering process from reporting to arrest. Even so, the number is still not nearly as high as in popular belief. Although it may be comforting for all concerned to simply blame the problem on drinking, it is much more complicated. Alcohol does provide the husband with a convenient excuse for his behaviour, or a denial of it, and it may be comforting for the woman to see the problem as caused by some extraneous factor beyond the relationship or outside of the husband's usual self. In all of these ways it plays a complex role in wife-beating, but it would be erroneous to accept the simplistic argument that the behaviour of men who beat their wives is simply dictated by drink.

UNDERSTANDING THE VIOLENCE AND THE
RESPONSES OF WOMEN

In studying the overall problem through the analysis of police records, in-depth interviewing and historical analysis, it became clear that a crucial factor in the generation of violence was the transition of single women into wives. Most women were subjected to violence only after they established a permanent relationship with the man who assaulted them. Their daily lives changed through marriage or permanent cohabitation, with increasing domestic labour, a diminished and restricted social life, and the man's increasing sense of rightful authority and possession, and with this they became subject to violence. Through marriage they were transformed into the 'appropriate' or 'legitimate' victims of rightful patriarchal chastisement.

We cannot over-stress the importance of the position and status of wives in the patterning of violence, and the importance of the man's sense of domination that accompanies marriage, as the most significant factors in wife-beating. Confrontations regarding the husband's authority and the wife's obligations to him become a persistent aspect of the relationship and provide a crucial factor in understanding violent events. Patriarchal patterns and the supporting ideology still prevail, and constitute the context in which wife-beating persists.

An important aspect of the patriarchal form of authority is a moral order emphasising obedience and loyalty of inferiors. Women are bound to the home not merely by domestic labour and child care, but also by a strong sense of moral responsibility for such tasks. Men are also somewhat bound by the demands of this moral order, but not nearly to the same degree as women. No matter how 'egalitarian' a relationship may be, it is the woman who is ultimately responsible for domestic work and child care. It is she who must arrange for baby-sitters or see that domestic work is done before she can go out, and even then she may be plagued by guilt since a 'good' mother must be constantly responsible for her household. Men, on the other hand, do not need to worry very much about such matters if they decide to go out for work or pleasure. The man who uses violence against his wife is often enforcing this moral order by punishing or correcting perceived failures to live up to the expectations of a 'good' wife and mother. The emotions and responses of women are also affected by ideals emphasising loyalty, obedience and domestic responsibility. Many of the women we interviewed felt guilty when their husbands attacked them, blamed themselves and kept the violence a secret.

This guilt can only be understood relative to social demands placing responsibility for a successful marriage primarily on women, and requiring wives to be loyal to their husbands regardless of their behaviour. Gradually, many women begin to question or reject this morality and their husbands' claims that the violence was caused by the woman's behaviour and was thus her fault. But the demand for loyalty and the placing of responsibility for marriages with women are powerful tools with which to keep a woman 'in her place', and reduce her challenges to her husband's authority. These ideals are deeply embedded in our historical legacy (Dobash and Dobash, 1979, 1981). Social, legal and religious institutions have traditionally promulgated a patriarchal order with the underlying tenets that loyalty and deference of subordinates are moral obligations, that patriarchy is a just and natural form of marriage, and challenges to it are defined as unacceptable and improper.

HELP-SEEKING

A battered woman's need for assistance from others, like the violence she experiences, begins early in the marital or cohabiting relationship and continues to change over time as the man's violence grows more frequent and severe and the woman actively seeks a cessation to it. Throughout this process a dynamic pattern develops which includes: the violence itself, the couple's overall relationship, the woman's contact with outsiders and the responses of those contacted. Violence, contacts and responses become inextricably intertwined in the development of the problem.

Patterns of help-seeking behaviour change over time and are related both to the severity of the violence and to the response of those approached for assistance. Based on the data from our interviews with battered women we will examine the pattern of help-seeking over time, particularly the contact between battered women and others. In brief, the evidence shows that: (1) seeking help from others is not solely related to the severity of an attack; (2) help-seeking is mediated through a number of social, moral and material factors relating to the woman's position as wife and mother within a patriarchal family structure; and (3) the nature of women's requests for help and the types of responses received from professionals and others change over time.

Although the literature on help-seeking behaviour is fairly extensive, there is little research on patterns of help-seeking among battered women. The majority of the work on help-seeking focuses either on the individual client or wider contextual factors (Brannen, 1980). The individual approach focuses on personal or psychological characteristics of clients, decision-making processes and/or knowledge and perception of services, while the contextual approach focuses on the social situation surrounding the client and the role of the agencies themselves. There is also some work using a more interactive perspective, focusing both on the clients and their relationship with the social agency. Regardless of the particular approach the results reveal that prospective clients usually have little knowledge about social agencies, and many have negative conceptions of them which lead to a reluctance to make and/or sustain contact (Weiss, 1973; Reith, 1975; Giordano, 1977). Overcoming this is very difficult and often affected by myth and rumour about the agency, the orientation of friends and relatives and the response of the agencies themselves (Nichols, 1976; Pahl, 1979; Brannen, 1980).

Our findings also show a reluctance to make contact either with informal sources such as relatives, friends or neighbours or with formal sources such as doctors, social workers and the police. Despite this, most women did make some form of contact on a few occasions, and very few women remained completely silent about the violence. While many women made an initial attempt to seek assistance, whether they continued to pursue such assistance often depended upon the response they received and the perceived effect the contact had on the cessation, continuation or escalation of the man's violent behaviour.

The changing nature of contacts is also apparent in the type of third party contacted. Women who made some type of contact after the first assault were most likely to go to informal sources, particularly relatives. Later they also approached formal sources, primarily doctors, social workers and the police. The reasons for this changing pattern of contacts are complex and relate to factors that vary over time. As we indicated above, after the first attack the women generally felt that they did not need assistance because the attack was seen as a unique event, which it was at the time, never to happen again. There was considerable hope for the future and little reason to believe otherwise. One woman remarked about the first assault, 'It never entered my head to go to anybody for help. I didn't need it. It was just an accident that could have happened to anyone at any time.' Men sometimes reinforced this, particularly after the first few attacks, by behaving in a contrite and apologetic manner and promising to reform. These interpretations and responses changed dramatically as the violence continued.

Examining why women do or do not seek help involves factors associated with the women, the men and the agencies themselves. One of the most important mechanisms inhibiting help-seeking for women is the shame and guilt associated with violence. Widely held beliefs about domestic privacy and autonomy, respectability and the notion that marital happiness and stability are the primary responsibility of women create feelings of shame and guilt and lead to silence. Violence often serves as an indicator to the woman that she has somehow 'failed', and for the violence to become public knowledge adds to this personal 'failure' and translates it into public stigma.

I felt very ashamed, very very ashamed, more ashamed than anything else and I certainly wouldn't let it be known to anybody, particularly my mother or the neighbours because I was supposed to be married and happy and to tell anybody would be nasty.

Since the family is perceived to be a private domain, it can be seen as wrong to breach this no matter how extreme the misbehaviour (Davidoff, L'Esperance and Newby, 1976; Elshtain, 1981; Pahl, 1985). The men often reinforced such ideals about privacy and contributed to the women's sense of shame, first by blaming them for 'provoking' the violence and then by maintaining that they deserved still more if the man's privacy and reputation were violated by seeking assistance from outsiders. In addition, patriarchal relationships are based upon belief in trust and loyalty from subordinates, and to seek outside help is a betrayal of this tacit bond of loyalty. This coercion of the conscience is a powerful mechanism in the arsenal of male domination.

Social and moral restraints were often accompanied by more direct physical barriers such as forcible confinement in the house and/or threatened reprisals. 'I wasn't allowed to a telephone box to phone the police or anybody. I wasn't allowed to get to the bleeding door, let alone the police.' Despite these obstacles, women certainly contemplated seeking assistance. But often, as with those who seek help for other types of problems, they did so with little knowledge of the agencies and considerable concern about the nature of the response they would receive. Many were afraid to seek help because they feared a negative response: 'My doctor's not the kind to give help or advice so I knew it was useless going to him. He was a man anyway and he would probably have sympathised with John [husband].' Some women did not wish to make contact because of a fear of intrusion into their family life and/or an increase in stigma: 'I felt that when you get in tow with these people [social workers] they interfere too much in your home life and with your kids, and the running of your house, which I didn't think was necessary.'

The woman's sense of isolation, shame and guilt, the man's justifications and threats, and concerns about negative responses did not, of course, completely prevent women from seeking help. They did contribute to considerable ambivalence and reticence about making and then maintaining contact. Over time, many of these impediments were outweighed as the frequency and intensity of the violence increased, and more and different kinds of assistance were sought. Indeed, it is important for professionals to recognise that it may not be the severity of a particular attack that leads a woman to seek help but rather the cumulative effect of persistent violence and intimidation, decreasing acceptance of the man's justifications and repeated failures to solve the problem alone. Despite this, the decision to approach a formal agency is a very difficult one and the initial contact so fraught with misgivings that the response can easily lead to a termination of contact.

REQUESTS AND RESPONSES

Despite the difficulties, most women eventually made some type of contact. The type of requests made and the responses received changed over time, and so did the degree of challenge each posed to the violence itself and to its social and ideological supports. Four general types of requests for assistance were made: (1) requesting assistance in stopping a particular attack; (2) seeking a sympathetic listener to give moral, medical or material support after an attack; (3) trying to involve others in the negotiations with the man in order to stop the continuing violence; and finally (4) attempting to gain the material assistance, such as accommodation and financial support, necessary to escape from a violent relationship. While the woman's particular requests varied in nature, they were all oriented in some way to trying to stop the violence.

An analytical examination of requests reveals that while all four types contain elements that could be defined as supportive of the woman, only three of them embody more direct and explicit challenges to the violence and/or its social underpinnings. For example, a woman may seek someone to talk to about the violence, and by doing so receive much-needed moral support and a lessening of isolation, but unless something else is done, sympathetic listening alone will not provide a direct challenge to the violence, whether it is a particular violent attack, the man's ongoing violent behaviour, the continuation of a violent relationship or the social relations that underpin and support wife-beating. Requests embodying challenges to the violence included attempts to gain assistance to stop a violent episode or remove it from the continuing relationship, as well as attempts to escape from a violent relationship.

The nature of the response may also be seen as potentially challenging the violence. In order to analyse this process we also characterised the responses as either supportive of the woman or challenging the violence. Supportive responses refer to those where, for example, the woman seeks a sympathetic listener and is heard, given credence and treated sympathetically, but no attempts are made to confront the violence itself. Challenging responses include such things as advising the woman about her rights and assisting her in obtaining them, trying to stop an attack in progress, speaking to the man about the unacceptability of his behaviour, referring to agencies and assisting the woman to escape from violence. Where the response was both supportive and challenging, it was defined as challenging. Although these two general characterisations of supportive and challenging actions were sufficient to define the women's requests, they were not sufficient for defining the responses. They also included a third type — negative actions such a denial, negation, victim-blaming and/or refusal to assist.

The nature of the requests made by the women changed over time from mostly supportive to mostly challenging. For example, after the first assault a total of 113 contacts were made with third parties and 73 per cent were requests for supportive forms of assistance. By comparison, a total of 371 contacts were made after the last assault and 66 per cent of them were for challenging forms of assistance.

The nature of the responses to supportive or challenging requests were diverse, ranging from attempts to minimise, deny or ignore them to active attempts to meet even the most challenging. Of course the nature of the response must be seen relative to the type of request made and the person to whom it was put. For example, relatives, particularly parents, were usually asked for both supportive and challenging types of assistance. Supportive requests were almost always responded to positively, and challenging ones, especially requests for temporary accommodation allowing escape for a few days, were usually, although certainly not always, met. Refusals were usually due more to problematic material circumstances limiting the ability to provide help than to a lack of willingness. 'I never wanted to go back but I was forced into it because me and the kids staying with Betty was just no use. She had her family to look after.' Friends and neighbours were more likely to be asked for supportive help than for challenging help, and these requests were usually met by friends but less frequently by neighbours.

Of the more formal groups, the medical profession rarely received challenging requests, whereas social services, housing departments and the police were often asked for such assistance. Obviously, statutory agencies have the resources and/or the sanctions that would be expected to provide meaningful challenges to the man's violence, while general practitioners do not: 'The doctor was helpful but there was nothing he could really do. He would just give you pills for your nerves and tell you it was up to you to sort things out.'

The responses of general practitioners were rather restricted and they rarely acted in a challenging way. Instead, they usually confined themselves to treating wounds, prescribing psychotropic medications and occasionally referring women to psychiatrists but rarely to other agencies. While most women told us that they initially appreciated medication, many eventually realised that it provided no solutions and might even exacerbate their predicament.

He put me on a course of tablets and I'd take the tablets and then would go back to see how the tablets helped and I'd tell him they did and I was fine. You weren't really telling lies because the tablets did help me but the same thing was happening again. I mean he was still hitting me. The tablets sort of calmed me down but they really didn't do much good.

Some very insensitive and unhelpful responses came from a few general practitioners:

I used to go round to the doctor's quite often because I couldn't sleep at night and my nerves were bothering me and I wasn't eating, but he just said, I can't help you while you're living with him; if he leaves or you leave him, come back and then maybe I'll be able to help you.

The doctor put me on drugs. He told me to get away and he asked me if I liked getting beaten up and I said 'No!!' and he said 'Well there must be something wrong with you because nobody could stand that much pain.'

Research in Britain and the United States reveals that some medical practitioners, like other social and legal professionals, think the problem is trivial, or that battered women are bad housewives, hysterical, masochistic, or actually like the violence (Cartwright, 1967; Rounsaville, 1977; Rounsaville and Weissman, 1977–78; Hilberman and Munson, 1978; Stark, Flitcraft and Frazier, 1979; Pahl, 1979; Binney et al., 1981). Such responses demonstrate a considerable failure to comprehend the predicament of battered women. Fortunately, not all general practitioners responded in these ways; some offered support and a few even attempted to challenge the husband with his culpability.

However, even seemingly helpful responses may sometimes increase the problem. For example, referral to and contact with a psychiatrist is likely to entail implicit, sometimes explicit, notions that the 'problem' resides in the woman's personality and/or behaviour. The long-standing psychiatric theories and professional ideologies emphasising the supposed provoking, masochistic and violence-seeking nature of women can result in victim-blaming (Snell, Rosenwald and Robey, 1964; Storr, 1974; Gayford, 1976; Shainess, 1977; Bowder, 1979; Pizzey and Shapiro, 1982). When these interpretations are coupled with the woman's existing feelings of shame they may exacerbate her predicament and reinforce her sense of guilt, while at the same time indirectly reinforcing the man's sense of justification.

The social and psychological predicaments of battered women are mainly invisible to the medical profession. They escape the medical gaze almost entirely, especially in the casualty ward (Stark et al., 1979; Women's Aid Federation, 1980). The one-way hierarchical nature of the medical examination which largely excludes dialogue makes it very unlikely that women will raise the problem, and general practitioners are also unlikely to do so. The general practitioner's failure to recognise or understand the problem must be understood relative to a background of patriarchal assumptions about women, institutional and situational demands made on the medical profession (too many patients, inadequate resources) and professional training that seeks to fit complex social, psychological and physical problems into neat, clear-cut physical symptoms defined as treatable within the context of medicine.

Social workers were usually asked for both supportive and challenging assistance. Challenging requests were usually for tangible assistance such as accommodation or resources that would enable the woman to leave. Women had greater expectations of social workers than of general practitioners. Yet it was the supportive requests rather than the challenging ones that were much more likely to be met.

One response that could be either supportive or challenging was casework counselling. However, this was rarely with the man, and could have a negative effect if it resulted in blaming the woman or otherwise making her responsible for solving the problem.

> I felt everybody was up against me, even socially. I felt inadequate as a woman. He was alright, he could do what he liked to me but nobody ever tried to help me. It seemed to me that the social workers and the doctors were blaming me for it.

> The social workers were sympathetic but it was always a case of, if he did that to me, I'd have done this to him and I'd have done that to him. So it was my fault, and I think they believed him.

There may be several reasons why social workers do not contact men and treat them as the party responsible for stopping the violence. Firstly, if the problem is seen primarily as the woman's this precludes the need to make contact with the man and also leads more easily to focusing on the woman as the source of the trouble. Secondly, many social workers may be intimidated by the idea of confronting a man known to be violent. This is also sometimes true of the police, who have much more experience in dealing with violent people. Thirdly, although some social workers did attempt to confront the man and/or actively pursue assistance for the woman, they acted primarily upon individual initiative and not because of priorities or policies set by the agency which would facilitate and legitimise such action.

The response of social workers generally reflected several concerns of fundamental importance to the profession: the protection and/or care of children, the maintenance of the family unit and the ideal of domestic privacy. The irony here is that while the mere suspicion of child abuse may result in swift action and intervention taking precedence over concern for family unity and domestic privacy, the certain knowledge of wife abuse rarely does so (Wilson, 1977; Dahl and Snare, 1978; Donzelot, 1980; Cavanagh, 1981). Many of the women we interviewed gave accounts of how their requests and need for assistance were relegated to a secondary position or ignored.

> I went to the welfare to get somewhere to stay but they couldn't help me. Mrs Jones [social worker] told me I would have to stay and I said, I just can't, and they said, You'll just have to stay for the sake of the wee ones. And at that stage I thought, My God all anybody can ever say to me is the wee ones, the wee ones,

but what about me?

> Once he [social worker] had made sure that the kids were in no danger he just went off and left me. And I thought, Huh, it seems nobody cares if I get beaten black and blue but if the kids do — which they weren't — then they get the attention I don't seem to deserve.

Maynard (1985) also found similar primacy in concerns for children and maintenance of the family unit in her examination of case notes of social workers. Her research revealed a general failure to focus on violence against wives along with an almost exclusive preoccupation with the welfare of children, the domestic skills of women and their supposed contribution to the violence. Furthermore, she found that while social workers apparently found it rather difficult to accept women's accounts of the violence, on the rare occasions when men were interviewed their rationalisations and condemnations of their wives appeared to have been given more credence than the women's. As one of the women we interviewed put it, 'Everybody seemed to think I was exaggerating every time I said anything about him.' In our study, social workers often advised women to simply cope with the violence and/or change their behaviour in order to appease their husbands.

> Patch it up. I thought I was going crackers with patch it up, patch it up, patch it up. . . . The Welfare all said to me . . . 'You've just got to stay in the home for the sake of the children. You've just got to keep the home together.' And of course there was little else I could do because they wouldn't help me to get a house or anything.

Such negative or unhelpful responses to battered women reflect several factors: statutory obligations to protect children but not women, numerous professional ideals about family unity and domestic privacy, psychoanalytic views of women, traditional orientations towards the relationships between men and women and the misguided concept of remaining 'neutral' (Nichols, 1976; Wilson, 1977; Pfouts, 1978; Schecter, 1982; Maynard, 1985). Regardless of the background to unhelpful, condemning or 'neutral' responses, the outcome often reinforces the man's domination and the woman's isolation and sense of guilt and shame. This, in turn, reduces the probability that continued assistance will be sought. In fact, negative or unhelpful responses were the main reasons given for not seeking further assistance from doctors, social workers and the police.

WOMEN'S AID REFUGES AND CHALLENGING MALE VIOLENCE

A social movement began in the early 1970s that has dramatically changed the persistent pattern of inadequate responses to battered women in Britain. Growing out of the women's movement, Women's Aid has provided thousands of women with direct assistance through the provision of refuges for battered women and their children (Charlton, 1972; Marcovitch, 1976; Hanmer, 1977; Sutton, 1978). They unequivocally rejected men's use of violence against women and provided numerous forms of assistance for battered women. There are now approximately 175 refuges in Britain associated with the Women's Aid Federations in Scotland, Wales, Northern Ireland and England. The federations explicitly adopt feminist principles and democratic forms of organisation in the operation of the national offices and in the running of refuges. The Women's Aid Movement does not, however, merely provide accommodation, it seeks to deal with women on their own terms and relative to their particular needs. Refuges provide the opportunity to meet and talk with other women who have experienced violence, provide support and advocacy from refuge workers and allow much-needed time to consider the future.

The work of the Women's Aid Movement has explicitly challenged the indifference and antagonism of many traditional responses to battering, that reflect patriarchal assumptions about women and men. This includes responses of social, legal and medical agencies that may condemn the violence, yet continue to accept and support the type of relationship that leads to it. It is important to identify such contradictory actions which implicitly or explicitly reject the violence while supporting its very foundations through attempting to excuse or justify the man's behaviour, by seeking provocation in the woman's behaviour or by viewing her as masochistic or 'violence-prone'. Perspectives of this nature usually lead to unhelpful forms of assistance.

In the past 10 years the problem of violence against women within the home has been placed on the public agenda in countries all over the world, and important support and protection has been provided by women through the work of groups such as Women's Aid. There have also been some legislative and administrative developments within housing and criminal justice. In Britain the Housing and Homeless Persons Act, the Domestic Violence and Matrimonial Proceedings Acts and the Domestic Proceedings and Magistrates Court Act were ostensibly designed to assist women to find housing and to provide better protection from violent men (Atkins and Hoggett, 1984). Unfortunately, these Acts have provided only limited support and protection for a few women. The problems are not so much in the specification of the Acts as in their interpretation and enforcement. Housing officials, magistrates and the police often still refuse to treat the problems of battered women seriously (Binney, Harkell and Nixon, 1981; Dobash and Dobash, 1981; Borkowski, Murch and Walker, 1983; Pahl, 1985). Recent research reveals that English magistrates rarely invoke the provisions of arrest provided for under the Domestic Violence Act (McCann, 1985) and housing officials fail to give women priority in housing needs (Binney *et al.*, 1981). It is still women in the community that provide the most significant support and advice for women. The professions — social work, medicine, housing and the police — have shown little initiative in dealing with the problem either at national or regional level, and have made few attempts to develop *systematic* forms of training that would equip these professionals to identify the problem and react effectively toward both the female victims and the male abusers. Importantly, male violence has not been confronted.

The future direction for institutional response is clear. Social workers, the police and other representatives of the social services must first examine their own beliefs and actions to determine how they may actually be contributing to the continuation of the violence, and the husband's sense of rightful control and violence must be explicitly and unequivocally rejected. We need to adopt a clearer and more straightforward view of, and response to, the problem, and replace indifference with a stance that more closely approximates that of the advocate. Organisational policies and practices must change so that rapid and supportive responses are frequent and easy, rather than exceptions requiring great time and effort from the highly motivated. We must attempt to confront the man and alter his sense of rightful authority and justification in using violence. This is not easy. Men who use violence do not believe they have a problem, and in many ways they do not since they are not the ones subjected to violence. It is also extremely important to respond to the problem as soon as possible after it appears, since men are more likely to feel guilt and wish to change in the beginning of a relationship.

The police should not continue to view the problem as one unworthy of their attention. They are mandated to enforce the law and protect the public, and this is what they should do regardless of the relationship between the victim and offender. In arresting the man who assaults his wife they will demonstrate to that husband and wife, and to other men and women, that violence against wives is an unacceptable and truly illegal behaviour. Indeed, research in the United States has now shown this to be the most effective police response (Sherman and Berk, 1984). This might be followed by alternative sanctions, instead of fines or prison. Alternative sanctions should focus on the man, not the woman or 'family', and include programmes for men to learn non-violent and non-destructive ways of relating to others such as those developed by 'Emerge' in Boston and 'Man Alive' in California (Emerge, no date; Man Alive, 1985). We also need a well-developed and widely publicised back-up and referral system, co-ordinating the efforts of medical practitioners, police, social work departments and Women's Aid refuges. Finally, the Women's Aid Federation and local refuges should be supported to the fullest, so that they can continue to provide the most tangible and important help for battered women. For over a decade they have provided vital accommodation and support for women. They have made great efforts to change public policy, social institutions and the wider society, directed both at responding effectively to those now experiencing violence and at eliminating it in the future.

ACKNOWLEDGEMENTS

This research was funded by a grant from the Scottish Home and Health Department. We would like to thank Jim Orford for his important contributions to the preparation of this chapter. We also acknowledge the Open University Press and Routledge & Kegan Paul for permitting us to use material from the following: Dobash, R.E. and Dobash, R.P. (1980) 'Wife Beating', in *Block III* (Abuse), p. 552, Open University Press, Milton Keynes; Dobash, R.E., Dobash, R.P. and Cavanagh, K., 'The Contact Between Battered Women and Social and Medical Agencies', in Pahl (ed.) *Private Violence and Public Policy*, Routledge & Kegan Paul, London.

REFERENCES

Atkins, S. and Hoggett, B. (1984) *Women and the law*, Basil Blackwell, Oxford

Binney,V., Harkell, G. and Nixon, J. (1980) *Refuge and housing for battered women in England and Wales*. Final report of the Women's Aid Federation/Department of the Environment Research Team

Binney, V., Harkell, G. and Nixon, J. (1981) *Leaving violent men: a study of refuges and housing for battered women*, Leeds, Women's Aid Federation (England)

Borkowski, M., Murch, M. and Walker, V. (1983) *Marital violence: the community response*, Tavistock, London

Bowder, B. (1979) The wives who ask for it, *Community Care*, 1 March, pp. 18–19

Brannen, J.A. (1980) Seeking help for marital problems: a conceptual approach, *British Journal of Social Work, 10*, 457–70

Cartwright, A. (1967) *Patients and their doctors*, Routledge and Kegan Paul, London

Cavanagh, K. (1981) The child abuse case conference: a feminist analysis Unpublished thesis, Department of Applied Social Studies, University of Warwick

Charlton, C. (1972) The first cow on Chiswick High Road, *Spare Rib, 24*, 24–5

Dahl, T.S. and Snare, A. (1978) The coercion of privacy: a feminist perspective. In C. Smart and B. Smart (eds), *Women, sexuality and social control*, Routledge and Kegan Paul, London

Davidoff, L., L'Esperance, J. and Newby, H. (1976) Landscape with figures. In J. Mitchell and A. Oakley (eds), *The rights and wrongs of women*, Penguin, Harmondsworth, pp. 139–75

Dobash, R.E. and Dobash, R.P. (1979) *Violence against wives: a case against the patriarchy*, Free Press, New York; Open Books, Shepton Mallet

Dobash, R.E. and Dobash R.P. (1984) The nature and antecedents of violent events, *British Journal of Criminology, 24*, 269–88

Dobash, R.P. and Dobash R.E. (1977) Wife beating, still a common form of violence, *Social Work Today, 9*, 14–19

Dobash, R.P. and Dobash, R.E. (1978) Wives: the 'appropriate' victims of marital violence, *Victimology, 2*, 426–72

Dobash, R.P. and Dobash, R.E. (1981) Community response to violence against wives: charivari, abstract justice and patriarchy, *Social Problems, 28*, 563–84

Dobash, R.P. and Dobash, R.E. (1983) The context specific approach to researching violence against wives. In G. Hotaling *et al.* (eds), *The dark side of families: current family violence research*, Sage, Beverly Hills, CA, pp. 261–76

Donzelot, J. (1980) *The policing of families*, Pantheon, New York

Elshtain, J.B. (1981) *Public man, private woman*, Martin Robertson, Oxford

Emerge (n.d.) A men's counselling service on domestic violence: an overview of services, *Emerge*, No. 206, 25 Huntington Ave., Boston, MA 02116, USA

Evason, E. (1982) *Hidden violence*, Farset Press, Belfast

Gaguin, D.A. (1978) Spouse abuse: data from the national crime survey, *Victimology, 2*, 632–43

Gayford, J.J. (1976) Ten types of battered wives, *Welfare Officer, 1*, 5–9

Gibson, E. (1975) *Homicide in England and Wales, 1967–71*, Home Office Research Study No. 31, HMSO, London

Gibson, E. and Klein, S. (1969) *Murder, 1957 to 1968*, a Home Office Statistical Division Report on Murder in England and Wales, HMSO, London

Giordano, P. (1977) The client's perspective in agency evaluation, *Social Work*, January, pp. 34–7

Hanmer, J. (1977) Community Action, Women's Aid, and the Women's Liberation Movement. In M. Mayo (ed.), *Women in the Community*, Routledge and Kegan Paul, London, pp. 91–108

Hilberman, E. and Munson, K. (1978) Sixty battered women, *Victimology*, 2, 460–70

McCann, K. (1985) Battered women and the law: the limits of legislation. In J. Brophy and C. Smart (eds), *Women in law*, Routledge and Kegan Paul, London

McClintock, E.H. (1963) *Causes of Violence*, St Martin's Press, New York

Man Alive (1985) Training Program for Men. Contact Hamish Sinclair, 345 Johnston Drive, San Rafael, California 94903, USA

Marcovitch, A. (1976) Refuges for battered women, *Social Work Today, 7*, 34–5

Maynard, M. (1985) The response of social workers to domestic violence. In J. Pahl (ed.), *Private violence and public policy*, Routledge and Kegan Paul, London

Nichols, B.B. (1976) The abused wife problem, *Social Casework, 57*, January, 27–32

Pahl, J. (1979) The general practitioner and the problems of battered women, *Journal of Medical Ethics, 5*(3), 117–23

Pahl, J. (1983) The allocation of money and the structuring of inequality within marriage, *Sociological Review, 31*, 2

Pahl, J. (1985) *Private violence and public policy*, Routledge and Kegan Paul, London

Pfouts, J.H. (1978) Violent families: coping responses of abused wives, *Child Welfare, LVII*, 101–11

Pizzey, E. and Shapiro, J. (1982) *Prone to violence*, Hamlyn, Feltham, Middlesex

Reith, D. (1975) I wonder if you can help me, *Social Work Today 6*, 66–9

Rounsaville, B.J. (1977) Battered wives, barriers to identification and treatment, *American Journal of Orthopsychiatry, 48*, 487–95

Rounsaville, B.J. and Weissman, M.M. (1977–78) Battered women: a medical problem requiring detection, *International Journal of Psychiatry in Medicine, 8*, 191–202

Schecter, S. (1982) *Women and male violence*, South End Press, Boston

Shainess, N. (1977) Psychological aspects of wife beating. In M. Roy (ed.), *Battered women: a psychological study of violence*, Van Nostrand Reinhold, New York, pp. 111–18

Sherman, L.W. and Berk, R.A. (1984) The specific deterrent effects of arrest for domestic assault, *American Sociological Review, 49*, 261–72

Snell, J.E., Rosenwald, R.J. and Robey, A. (1964) The wife-beater's wife, *Archives of General Psychiatry, 11*, August, 107–12

Stark, E., Flitcraft, A. and Frazier, W. (1979) Medicine and patriarchal violence, *International Journal of Health Services, 9*, 461–93

Storr, A. (1974) *Human aggression*, Penguin Books, Harmondsworth

Sutton, J. (1978) The growth of the British movement for battered women, *Victimology, 2*, 576–84

Voss, H.L. and Hepburn, J.R. (1968) Patterns in criminal homicide in Chicago, *Journal of Criminal Law, Criminology and Police Science, 59*, 499–508

Wasoff, F. (1982) Legal protection from wife beating: the processing of domestic assaults by Scottish prosecutors and criminal courts, *International Journal of Sociology of Law, 10*, 187–204

Weiss, R. (1973) Helping relationships: relations of clients with physicians, social workers, priests and others, *Social Problems, 20*, 187–204

Wilson, E. (1977) *Women and the welfare state*, Tavistock, London

Wolfgang, M.E. (1958) *Patterns in criminal homicide*, Wiley, New York

Women's Aid Federation (England) (1980) An abnormal number of malevolent doorknobs: battered women and the medical profession, a preliminary survey. London Women's Aid Federation

Worrall, A. and Pease, K. (1986) Personal crime against women: evidence from the British Crime Survey, *Howard Journal of Criminal Justice, 25*, 118–124

9

Depression and the Family

Liz Kuipers

Some days he's just awful. I feel I offer my crumbs of support when I can. If I gave it all, the marriage would be over in a few months (wife about her husband).

Depression is a major problem for the community. The lifetime expectancy of contacting a psychiatric hospital with depression may be as high as 11 per cent for men and 20 per cent for women (Sturt, Kumakura and Der, 1984). Nor is it a problem which leads only to short periods of disability. In many cases the problem becomes a chronic one. Mann and Cree (1976), in a study of 'new long-stay' hospital patients aged between 18 and 65, found that affective psychosis accounted for 15.8 per cent of patients, and that they formed the largest single group after schizophrenia.

Despite this there is surprisingly little known specifically about the families of depressed people. Research that has been carried out has not concentrated on this diagnostic grouping, and many of the findings relate to relatives of all discharged psychiatric patients and must be inferred for this particular group. The evidence which does exist suggests that the effect of this disorder and its impact on family members can be every bit as devastating as for more debilitating psychiatric disorders such as schizophrenia.

Typically, the closest relatives involved with a depressed person are spouses or cohabitees. Despite general figures showing lower marriage and fertility rates for those with psychiatric disorders, as well as higher divorce rates (Slater, Hare and Price, 1971), these are most extreme in schizophrenia, and depressed people in contact with a relative are likely to be married, and many have children. The literature on effects on relatives is thus not only scant but it also deals exclusively with the effects on spouses and to some extent on children.

MODELS

There are two main models and a subsidiary one which have been described and investigated in relation to depressed patients and their families. I shall term them the interactional, the stress or adversity, and the reactive models.

The interactional model

Because relatives are primarily partners, attention has been focused on the marriages of depressed people. There has been interest in discovering whether some marriages are 'depressogenic', themselves causing depressive symptomatology. There is certainly evidence to support the view that negative interactions and a poorer quality of marriage are associated with depression in one of the partners. More extreme exponents of this model suggest that such marriages not only maintain but produce depressive symptomatology. Hinchliffe, Hooper and Roberts (1978) have coined the term 'the melancholy marriage', and in an observational study showed higher levels of negative communication in couples with a depressed partner, compared with couples with a surgically ill partner, or compared with the depressed partner talking to a neutral person. They have used this as evidence for the causal role of the system. Crammer (1971) has classified constructive and destructive responses of spouses and other family members to the depressed patient at home. Feldman (1976) has described ways in which a partner may maintain or trigger depressive symptomatology by remarks which undermine a patient's self-worth. Kreitman (1964), in a study of the spouses of depressed psychiatric patients, found they were more likely to be neurotic and had more physical and psychological symptoms than control subjects. He has suggested that the neurotic patient operates interactionally within a shrinking social framework which normally involves a spouse. The partners then become increasingly involved with each other and tend to become more alike. Assortative mating is not supported because there is little evidence to differentiate depressed patients from their spouses or controls at the beginning of the marriage. These findings have been confirmed in a larger study (Kreitman, Collins, Nelson and Troop, 1970).

The quality of the marriage has also come under scrutiny. Rutter and Quinton (1977) found depressed or neurotic women to be five times as likely to have a disturbed marriage as normal women.

Weissman and Paykel (1974), in an American study of women, looked at some interactional features of the depressed woman's marriage both at the time of the illness and at the time of recovery. They describe the damaging effects of friction and hostility which may occur between the wife and the rest of the family during the illness, and which may then become difficult to reverse as the illness recedes. They discuss the possibility that these effects may be associated with poor pre-illness relationships as well as being one result of the illness process. Birtchnell and Kennard (1983) have presented data from three surveys suggesting that the quality of marriage exerts a powerful influence upon the depressive symptomatology of the women studied, and discuss the role of dependency in these marriages. Other factors which have been described in marriages with a depressed partner are more frequent conflicts over role function (Ovenstone, 1973); increasing pathology in the husband which is associated with less joint decision-making (Collins, Kreitman, Nelson and Troop, 1971) and reduced independent social activity of wives of depressed men compared to controls (Nelson, Collins, Kreitman and Troop, 1970).

The stress or adversity model

The second model posits that stress or adversity is associated with depression. It takes several forms, but they all suggest that depressed people are sensitive to stress in immediate relationships and the environment.

The most obvious stresses are life events, and it has been reported that depressed people are particularly responsive to them (Brown and Harris, 1978; Bebbington, Hurry and Tennant, 1981), and are not protected against life stresses by maintenance treatment (Paykel and Tanner, 1976; Paykel, 1978). Life events involving interpersonal arguments have been found to be most stressful (Jacobs, Prusoff and Paykel, 1974; Billings, Cronkite and Moos, 1983). Brown, Bhrolchain and Harris (1975) showed in a Camberwell sample that 30 per cent of women without a close confiding relationship developed psychiatric symptoms which were predominantly depressive when exposed to a severely stressful life event or major difficulty, but that only 4 per cent of those with a confidant did. There is also some evidence that life events precipitate manic episodes (Leff, Fischer and Bertelsen, 1976; Ambelas, 1979; Kennedy, Thompson, Stancer, Roy and Persad, 1983).

Research on the factor of expressed emotion (EE) has shown that this is not just associated with relapse in schizophrenic patients with families. Vaughn and Leff (1976) included a group of 30 depressed neurotic patients in their sample, and found that they were also sensitive to the critical remarks of their spouses and liable to become ill in the next year. Indeed this appeared to be so at even lower levels of criticism than was the case for schizophrenic patients. This finding has been replicated recently by Hooley and her colleagues (Hooley, Orley and Teasdale, 1985).

The role of criticism in exacerbating depressive symptomatology is also supported by a small study of people experiencing mania, showing that interpersonal conflicts need to be avoided if relapse is to be prevented (Lieberman and Strauss, 1984).

The reactive model

Another perspective on families with a depressed member is contained in a reactive model. Unlike the other two models this does not, either implicitly or explicitly, imply any causal mechanisms, but rather looks at family reactions to the problems of living with a depressed person. Mental health professionals tend to assume pathology, rather than normal behaviour which may be distorted by unusual or bizarre circumstances. The factors that have been identified as associated with depressive symptomatology in families — poor marriage, negative communications, interpersonal conflicts and an unsympathetic atmosphere at home — could all be seen as reactions on the part of a spouse to depression in a partner. These reactions may well make things worse, but have become part of rigid and dysfunctional patterns of behaviour that neither partner can easily change.

All these models fail to explain some aspects of depression in families. The interactional model tends to imply causal factors in the behaviour of the partner for which there is no conclusive evidence. Nor does it encompass families which do not show negative factors but which still contain a depressed member. The stress model concentrates on triggering factors and on the depressed patient's sensitivity to the environment. It does not explain depressive episodes not connected to environmental events. The reactive model says nothing about causes or how a first depression begins. However its advantage is that it tries to assume normal and understandable responses in relatives rather than exacerbating the blame and guilt that relatives often feel.

It is probable that all three viewpoints need to be considered as they are by no means mutually exclusive. The reactive model in particular has not been generally emphasised, and it may be timely to do so, not only to enhance more positive professional attitudes towards families, but also to enable a better understanding and appreciation of the problems that relatives may face and the burden they may carry when living with a depressed spouse at home.

THE IMPACT OF DEPRESSION ON THE FAMILY

Very few studies have looked specifically at depression in terms of the impact on the family or the burden it imposes. This section will be divided into two parts. The first part will look at studies which included some depressed psychiatric patients but which comment on the general problems of living with the mentally ill. These are relevant because many of the problems overlap with those found in families with patients in other diagnostic categories, particularly if the problems persist. The second part will concentrate on the few specific studies which have looked at depressed people and the impact of the disorder on their spouses and children.

General effects of living with a person who is mentally ill

The first studies of the sorts of demands on families that could be expected when a mentally ill hospital patient returned home were carried out in the mid-1950s by a group of social scientists in the United States (Clausen, Yarrow, Deasy and Schwartz, 1955; Yarrow, Schwartz, Murphy and Deasy, 1955). They studied 33 families where the husband was a patient with a diagnosis of psychosis or psychoneurosis. Hence several of the families must have suffered from depression. The investigators followed the wife's reaction from the time of her husband's first admission to hospital, to 6 months after his return home or to the end of his first year of hospitalisation. The findings pinpoint a number of important problem areas, which are confirmed by later studies. First there was a difficulty in deciding which behaviour was 'normal', or 'not normal', because of the overlap of many symptoms with ordinary patterns of behaviour. Wives tended to attribute problems to character defects in their husbands such as 'weakness' or 'a lack of willpower'.

Secondly, the husband's illness had a noticeable impact on the wife's social relationships. Because of the stigma of mental illness many wives cut off former relationships and tried to conceal their husbands' problems. Thirdly, wives felt an impact on themselves. There were feelings of guilt and blame in case they or the relationship had caused the problems. Many wives experienced anxiety and feelings of rejection towards their husbands. Several had contemplated separation or divorce.

Finally the researchers examined the relationships between the wives and their husbands' psychiatrists and the attitudes that each held towards the other (Deasy and Quinn, 1955). The majority of requests by wives were for information about the illness, and advice on how to deal with the patient when he returned home. However most wives expressed dissatisfaction because they did not receive such information, or doctors were innaccessible. The psychiatrists' point of view was different. Although they viewed it as reasonable to provide information, they did not necessarily see it as their job, thought it too time-consuming, and did not always feel able to answer questions because of the nature of mental illness and its uncertainties. There was also the finding that psychiatrists frequently felt they had to protect the patient from his wife since factors in the husband-wife relationship had contributed to the husband's illness.

Thus at this early stage key problem areas were highlighted: the problems of differentiating illness behaviour from normal behaviour and thus being able to understand or tolerate it; the psychological impact of the illness on the spouse; the reduced social network that is imposed by stigma; the problem of communicating with mental health professionals. Those four problems remain today, in both depressive and other disorders.

The first study to look in detail at the different areas of people's lives which are affected when a mentally ill relative lives at home was by Mills (1962), who interviewed 76 patients with various diagnoses, and 74 relatives. Practically all of the patients caused anxiety to their relatives, with over half being described as 'difficult'. One concern was that the patient might be a danger to him/herself or others. Another was the problems caused with neighbours because of the patient's behaviour. Many relatives had disturbed nights, but found things like apathy or withdrawal more difficult than the practical problems. The patient's illness also caused financial problems and a restricted social life for the family.

Similar findings were reported by Grad and Sainsbury (1963), again with a general group of psychiatric patients, some of whom would have been suffering from depression. These researchers attempted to rate the burden that these families described using a three-point scale. They reported effects on the family such as income reduction, restriction of social and leisure activities, disruption of domestic routine, disturbances in children, and neurotic symptoms including anxiety, depression, insomnia and irritability in the spouses and parents of the patients. Again, the problems which relatives found most difficult to cope with were not the violent or socially embarrassing behaviour usually associated with mental illness, but things such as depressive ruminations and hypochondriacal preoccupations that patients exhibited.

Hoenig and Hamilton (1966, 1969) distinguished between objective burden (such as financial loss) and subjective burden (the extent to which relatives felt burdened). In their study of variously diagnosed discharged hospital patients, 76 per cent of patients had produced some kind of adverse effect for the household. These included general disruption of family life, financial difficulties and health effects on other family members. Once again extreme withdrawal was found more difficult to cope with than aggressive behaviours. The duration of the illness was also found, not surprisingly, to be an important factor, with objective burden likely to be greater for a family the longer an illness persisted. There were also interesting differences between objective and subjective burdens, with many families tolerating high levels of burden, and few expecting services to provide any help.

Finally Creer, Sturt and Wykes (1982) carried out a survey of the relatives of the long-term mentally ill in which about one-third suffered from some sort of affective disorder, and about 40 per cent lived at home with relatives. They found that relatives were coping with very difficult behaviour at home, the same sorts of things that staff in hospital were dealing with, but with little support and no specific professional group concerned with relatives' needs, as professionals remain primarily patient-oriented. The main requirements of relatives were for information and practical advice, for emotional support, and occasional breaks or holidays.

Thus from these studies, which all included some patients with depressive disorders, the following factors, highlighted by Clausen and colleagues 30 years ago, emerge consistently:

1. The difficulties relatives have in understanding that behaviour may be caused by the illness when it overlaps with ordinary behaviour patterns. The so-called 'negative' symptoms, the loss of behaviours, are the ones most likely to cause this confusion — things like loss of interest, apathy, loss of conversation skills, not getting up in the morning, lack of interest in self-care. If these behaviours are

not understood then family members find it harder to tolerate them.

2. The psychological impact of the illness on the spouse; effects can include guilt, anxiety and rejection of the partner.
3. The financial problems of families and their reduced social network and social activities.
4. The lack of support from mental health professionals.

Specific effects of living with depression

The key finding from the small amount of research on families coping with depression is that they are characterised by impaired communications. This is usually negative, consisting of things such as reduced eye contact, slowed speech, and less humour (Hinchliffe et al., 1978) and may be accompanied by high levels of tension, quarrelling and disharmony (Weissman and Paykel, 1974). Typically the patient's spouse receives less affection and warmth from the patient. Performance in household tasks is likely to be reduced. Where impaired communication and affection does exist it is reported to have a much greater impact on the family than symptom behaviour itself (Vaughn and Leff, 1981). A distinction has also been made in terms of whether the patient happens to be male or female. Wives are typically reported to become more dependent and desirous of continual comfort and support which, of course, cannot always be supplied (Vaughn and Leff, 1981; Birtchnell and Kennard, 1987). Husbands, on the other hand, have been reported as being more likely to be socially withdrawn.

The impairment in communication is likely to be linked specifically with depressed symptomatology as it is reported to improve as the illness recedes, although some long-term negative effects can still be seen after recovery (Weissman and Paykel, 1974). It is not by any means the only effect that a depressive disorder can have on the family. A small, recent study of the relatives of 24 depressed patients (Fadden, Bebbington and Kuipers, 1985) set out to investigate specifically the effects on spouses of living with a depressed patient.

The findings with respect to the impact of the disorder fall into three categories: the objective burden; the types of symptoms relatives found difficult; and the psychological effects on relatives. Eight of the patients had a bipolar disorder, and the others had a neurotic or severe unipolar depressive disorder, all of several years duration, so that problems were all long-term.

The practical consequences of the illness confirm the earlier research. Two-fifths of the relatives (41 per cent) said that the state

201

of their finances was much worse since the patient became ill. The majority of the relatives (71 per cent) had experienced a reduction in social activities; wives were more likely to be affected than husbands. Because of the social isolation most families spent a lot of time together (an average of 65 hours per week). This finding has not arisen before and may not be general, but suggests that for this group relatives really were the primary care agents.

Many couples reported difficulties in the relationship, particularly the wives in the neurotic and unipolar depression group. These difficulties referred to loss of affection, sexual contact, and of their own support. Half of the couples had no children, and this was more often the case when the patients were female.

The problem behaviours reported were primarily sleep disturbance, followed by misery, underactivity, worry, fearfulness, irritability, social withdrawal, slowness and overdependence. Predictably the more florid behaviours were *less* likely to be seen as problems, as they appear to be more obviously due to an illness and thus more understandable. Thus the most florid group, the manic depressive group, were easier to tolerate in some ways than the neurotically depressed patients, who were likely to have symptoms that relatives thought patients could control.

The psychological effects on the relatives were again most marked in the neurotic depressed group. Feelings of loss and a changed relationship, together with grief, guilt and sorrow, were common reactions. Many had felt like separating. The depressed family members were described as behaving like children and thus being more demanding, dependent and not providing the spouses with their own adult support.

Many relatives felt that *they* had had to change. Some now responded differently to the spouse. Some had had to become more assertive and independent and take over roles in the family. Wives in particular did not always welcome these changes in role, and did not always relish having to become the breadwinners. Others felt things had deteriorated, particularly in the neurotic and unipolar group. Over a third were rated on a psychiatric interview as being psychiatrically ill themselves; the expected rate of such illness would be around 10 per cent.

One family, where the husband had a 5-year history, talked of the strain on the wife and their 10-year-old daughter. It was hard to explain to the child that she must be careful what she said to her father; if she happened to call him 'stupid' or 'silly' at the beginning of the day, he would be unable to leave the house. The wife felt very much that she was without support for herself and, while she tried to be sympathetic, often found herself becoming resentful and angry with her husband. This would make the situation worse and deepen her husband's self-doubt, inactivity and silences. She was committed to maintaining the marriage but felt that this was now becoming much more difficult, and that her own health was suffering.

Thus again the specific effects of a depressive illness on a family centre on problems in communication, leading to a loss of support and affection for the spouse while more roles have to be taken on. There is a greater likelihood that the ill partner will show dependent, childlike behaviour and will keep asking for reassurance. The behaviours that seem most difficult are the ones that are not recognisable as due to an illness, so that the neurotically depressed group may be the hardest to understand and their behaviour least likely to be tolerated by relatives. The psychological effects on spouses centre on stigma, loss and the stress of living in this situation, and are associated with neurotic disorders occurring in previously well relatives.

Effects on children

Partly because there is reduced fertility in psychiatric disorders, including depression, this question has also been little researched, and particularly so for this diagnosis. There is some evidence, however, that repeated depressive episodes or long-lasting depressive behaviours do have major effects on children (Hinchliffe *et al.*, 1978).

Rutter (1966) has pinpointed repeated disruption as the most important factor leading to suffering and disturbance in a child, not separation itself. Rutter also emphasises that the quality of maternal care is more important than the quantity. Continuity of care by the other parent or a surrogate figure is desirable. Because long-term psychiatric illness, particularly depression as has been noted, is often associated with chronic marital conflict, this can both exacerbate the symptoms of the patient and be a powerful influence in disturbing the family as a whole. Persistent neurotic disorder apparently has a greater effect than recurrent psychotic illness. Rutter has also noted differences in individual children's susceptibilities to living with mental illness. Boys appear to be more vulnerable than girls and produce higher levels of overt neurotic and anti-social behaviour. The levels of disturbance in children are likely to be greater where both parents are disturbed and there is less chance of continuous high-quality care being received by the child.

There is also evidence that the effects of the reduced non-verbal and emotional responses of depressed mothers on young children can lead to later problems unless they can be compensated for. Lomas (1967) has suggested that depression in a parent can lead to a poor psychological environment for a child due to inadequate physical contact with the child; the diminished ability of a parent to understand reality; the lack of emotional response in a parent which will discourage a child from expressing or receiving emotion; and lack of a good model for ordinary patterns of behaviour.

To summarise, the effects of a depressive disorder on the families living with a depressed member are concentrated on spouses and the marital relationship itself. While some relationships remain intact, and some spouses unaffected, there are likely to be changes, and these seem to centre on impaired communication, reduced support and role changes which may not be welcomed. Financial loss and increased social isolation are likely. Professional support may be lacking or unhelpful. This leaves many spouses in an unenviable position, and reports of neurotic disorders and their own feelings of stress are not surprising. What is interesting is how many spouses stay in the relationship and attempt to cope with these problems.

The effects on children are not specifically documented for this group but it is noted that long-term disruption and poor quality of care are the main factors likely to lead to later distress and behaviour problems in children. It has been suggested that, if alternative care can be provided by the other parent or another concerned adult, this may be very helpful. While this seems likely, there is no real evidence as yet to determine whether alternative care can protect or insulate children from such problems.

WAYS THAT FAMILIES DO COPE

There are only two studies in the literature which have addressed this issue at all. The research by Vaughn and Leff on the relatives of 30 depressed, neurotic, out-patients (1976) also analysed their interactions and the content of any critical remarks made. They concluded that the major determinant of a relative's response to the patient and the illness was the way the patient and relative related to each other *before* the illness started. Thus if the pre-illness relationship was good then the relative was either concerned and not critical, or critical but only of the patient's florid symptoms. However, the majority of relatives had a poor pre-illness relationship which had been characterised by major strain and disharmony and markedly impaired communication. In these cases, of course, the illness exacerbated the situation. Also in these cases the relatives tended to be critical of their spouses and their characteristics; many doubted that their partners were ill at all and described their partners' symptoms as an exaggeration of their normal behaviour, which they should try to control. One coping response in this situation, particularly for male partners, was avoidance and minimal contact.

Fadden *et al.* (1987) looked specifically at relatives' coping responses. Coping strategies varied: 92 per cent wished the situation would go away; 58 per cent agreed that 'they looked for the silver lining'. One-third criticised or lectured themselves, another third ate or drank more. Nearly half stated that they had *no idea what to do*. Two-thirds could not see things from the depressed person's viewpoint. Three-quarters reported that they did not discuss the situation with anyone or try to find out more about the problems. Half hoped that the patient would be 'cured' one day, and kept going.

These results suggest that relatives coped day to day with problems as they arose, tried not to think about the future and had no informed idea of what strategies were helpful, what they should be aiming at, or what the patient felt. As a group they were isolated from support, as has become clear, and were not receiving advice about management. Strategies which existed mainly concerned changing the individual, trying to reduce the relative's own stress and hoping that things would change.

The only evidence for familial responses that help in these situations comes from the work on expressed emotion (EE), with low EE, or less critical, spouses being associated with low relapse rates in depressive disorders (Vaughn and Leff, 1976; Hooley *et al.*, 1985). Characteristics of these low EE families suggest, first, that believing the patient to be ill is essential. If a relative is able to separate illness-related behaviour from 'normal' behaviour then the former becomes more understandable and easier to cope with. Understanding things from the patient's point of view is part of this process, and relatives who can manage this to some extent appear to be at an advantage. Secondly, being able to tolerate difficult behaviour appears helpful. Lowered expectations of performance and an assumption that the patient is not necessarily in control of his or her own behaviour, that silences, misery, worrying and no housework are not aimed at the spouse personally, and are upsetting for the patient too, help this kind of attitude. Thirdly, a sympathetic and caring approach to the patient, which is easier to maintain if the pre-illness relationship has been good, is an advantage.

As the evidence for depressive disorders suggests that becoming ill again is associated with even quite low levels of criticism, it seems likely that the patient is unusually sensitive to an unsympathetic atmosphere. It can be surmised that a depressed patient with already low levels of self-esteem or self-worth, negative thoughts, feelings of guilt and slowed responses or worrying, will be liable to be responsive to anything which exacerbates this state, and thus that any improvements in these areas, and in the support which a spouse can give, will be beneficial for the patient.

POINTERS TO THE HELP WHICH FAMILIES NEED

For 30 years families have consistently identified at least some of the areas in which they would like help. Obviously in this field identifying such needs has not guaranteed widespread professional responses to meet them. The most basic requirements of relatives which they themselves ask for are, first, information about the depressive disorder. Confusion exists in many families about differentiating illness behaviour from other behaviour. It is not always clear to relatives which behaviour the patient could be expected to exert control over and which they might need help with. Thus information about negative symptoms, the lack of behaviour, the slowness of response, poor performance in household and other tasks, and difficulties in interacting socially, would be particularly relevant. 'Educating' relatives in this sort of way has had some impact in reducing unsympathetic attitudes amongst relatives of people suffering from schizophrenia (Berkowitz, Eberlein-Fries, Kuipers and Leff, 1984), although there are problems with didactic material and an interactional approach is indicated, as otherwise people do not take in new and unfamiliar material (Tuckett, 1982).

Secondly, relatives continue to ask for advice about management of problem behaviours. The feeling seems to be that professionals know how to handle difficulties but either assume that the relative does not have to cope with the same problems, or do not think it is their particular profession's job to spend time discussing it. The other possibility, of course, is that professionals do not know what to advise. In many cases there are helpful management suggestions that could be discussed with relatives. Generally aims and expectations about future outcomes and performance could be made more explicit; for instance the fact that changes may be quite slow and need to be taken in stages, that improvements may take weeks or months rather than days. Specific advice about, say, how to get a patient out of bed in the mornings is available; a firm but tolerant approach, encouraging rather than nagging, reminders accompanied by a cup of tea but not breakfast, plus something positive to get up for, have all been found to work by other relatives (Kuipers and Bebbington, 1985).

Thirdly, although most relatives do not complain, the amount of care they often have to give, the unremitting nature of living with a depressed spouse and the lack of other social outlets, have led consistently to relatives wanting an occasional break or holiday from the depressed person. This suggests that social admissions to hospital or other residential care for this reason should not be ruled out. Groups concerned with the care of other disorders have organised this for themselves or through social services, but this has not happened for depressed people's relatives, as yet.

Other pointers exist which are identifiable from the literature. The financial problems of families with a depressed member are a consistent finding. Presumably because the depressed person living with a family is likely to be a joint head of a household, either being the main earner or providing house and child-care, and because these functions and performance are likely to be disrupted by a depressive illness, a drop of income is very likely to accompany onset, and is a factor for many families. While it is not the aim of most professional help to alleviate this problem it would seem useful that professionals be aware that financial difficulties might exist, and then to point relatives towards a Citizen's Advice Bureau or a social work department so that help can be offered to maximise the take-up of benefits that do exist.

Social isolation is another factor frequently identified as a problem due to stigma, the difficulties of explaining unusual behaviour in a spouse, the lack of social activities, and the demanding nature of the illness which can lead to relatives feeling 'smothered' by the depressed partner. Reduced finances will also be likely to make it more difficult to expand social or leisure activities. In other disorders self-help groups have been set up to answer this problem, and to begin to provide an alternative and supportive social network. They are also indicated for this disorder. The only one so far in existence is Depressives Associated.

Finally marital help, or help with the relationship of the depressed partner, is indicated, given the amount of disharmony, strain, poor quality of marriage, negative communication patterns, and unsympathetic attitudes that have all been found associated with a depressive disorder, and which are certainly exacerbated by a depressive disorder if they existed before its onset. The aims of such help would be primarily to improve the communication pattern and make it more positive. Whether it is causal or the result of the depressive illness, communication difficulty is one of the most noticeable features of a depressed person's relationship, and is likely to be causing some problems in about two-thirds of marriages. Another aim would be to enable the partner to recognise and tolerate more of the depressed person's behaviour, hence reducing unsympathetic, critical and uncaring attitudes on the part of the spouse. A final aim would be to improve performance; to encourage and build up behaviour patterns that had been lost or slowed by the depression, to help increase competence and the number of practical things the person could do, and also to help improve self-image and worth. Currently such specialist help is only available in a very few centres.

WHAT TREATMENTS ARE EFFECTIVE?

While there is evidence that the individual treatment of depression can ameliorate the condition, particularly if a combination of drug therapy and cognitive therapy is offered (Teasdale, 1985), evidence for the effectiveness of family, or specifically in this case marital, treatment is mainly descriptive or limited to small numbers. Hinchliffe *et al.* (1978) advocate and offer marital therapy for depressed couples. They emphasise the interactional nature of the disorder, backed by their own research, and advocate the use of General Systems Theory as a model for intervention. They see depression, 'in terms of the nature and quality of the interaction which surrounds the person who is labelled as the patient' (p. 84).

Hinchliffe *et al.* provide frequent case examples to describe in detail methods that can be used, and the sorts of problems that emerge. Marital therapy is the obvious mode in which a systems approach is used, but they agree that in some instances it may not be possible or desirable to see both spouses together, and individual sessions with the patient's partner may be indicated as well as joint sessions. One of the main aims of conjoint therapy is 'to actually facilitate and enlarge the spouse's sense of being able to be helpful' (p. 98). They suggest that one can intervene by interpreting spouses' needs to each other, and that spouses should be encouraged to express their real feelings towards their partners and to be aware of the hazards of assuming a tense, emotion-free posture. They try to identify and break down dysfunctional negative communication patterns and to replace them with more positive interactions. Other problems, such as letting the depressed partner take on more roles in the relationship again, and the function of the depressed patient's behaviour in the family system, are highlighted.

The main evidence that Hinchliffe and her co-workers cite as showing positive results for conjoint marital therapy is not their own work but an American study by Friedman (1975). This was a large and complex study which looked at many factors and used multiple-outcome measures. Friedman and his team conducted a trial of a 12-week course of treatment for 196 depressed out-patients, 166 of whom attended for treatment. Subjects were both male and female, but predominantly the latter. He compared drug plus marital therapy, drug plus individual therapy with minimal therapeutic contact, placebo plus marital therapy, and placebo plus minimal contact. Thus there was no control for the amount of therapeutic time spent on the marital therapy. The minimal contact consisted of half an hour per fortnight, whereas the marital therapy consisted of one hour per week, so that it may have been the case that it was not the content of the marital therapy but the frequency and amount of treatment which was more effective. Friedman reported no special difficulties in compliance in the marital therapy group.

The drug plus marital treatment condition resulted in improvements in symptoms after 12 weeks, compared to the placebo or minimal contact only conditions. Marital therapy improved self-report ratings on family roles and tasks compared to active drug treatment. Measures of marital relations were rated as worse in the marital therapy group, suggesting that depressed spouses had learned to assert themselves more against their partners. However as the improvements for each treatment condition also varied depending at which point in time the measurements were made, it is hard to pinpoint any more consistent findings for each treatment.

Friedman concluded that, 'for most of the outcome measures, the patient group that received both active drug and marital therapy showed more improvement, though not always to a statistically significant degree, than any of the other three patient groups' (p. 636). Overall the global improvement rates were 75 per cent improved, 19 per cent no change and 6 per cent worse, which suggests that the study as a whole was effective even in the minimal contact conditions. Unfortunately there are no follow-up data so that information about the efficacy of this large and well-designed trial is limited to the 12 weeks of its duration. There is also no clear description of what took place in the marital sessions, so that although Hinchliffe *et al.* claim its results support their ideas, it may be that the methods and orientation were not at all similar. Nevertheless it remains an important paper, suggesting that some interventions can be effective with this group, at least in the short term.

In contrast to this study, Rush, Shaw and Khatami (1980), also working in the USA, present only three case examples. However this group have been interested in the application of the use of cognitive therapy with selected depressed patients and their partners, which is an innovative use of this therapy. Rush *et al.* maintain that 'spouse involvement appears to alter the tendency of the couple to ascribe problems in the relationship to presumed defects in the depressed person' (p. 111). The techniques of cognitive therapy consist of verbal and behavioural methods designed to help a patient become aware of, and test against reality, selected distorted thinking patterns and idiosyncratic beliefs that form the basis of depressed cognitions. These techniques are used to address particular target symptoms such as pessimism, inactivity and guilt, and to modify specific thinking patterns, such as over-generalisation and selective attention to the negative, which accompany depressed behaviour. Behavioural practice between sessions is also encouraged.

In this study it is claimed that the participation of both spouses may facilitate cognitive change by providing a forum where a spouse acts as an information source or offers alternative views that provoke the patient to reconsider conceptualisations of self, the relationship, and the world at large. The couples format allows the therapist to directly observe and correct interpersonal behaviours that may maintain depressed, distorted thinking. Thus the role of the partner was to enable destructive interactive sequences to be observed and discussed, to help provide another disconfirming view of the depressed partner's negative cognitions, and to act as an ally in the therapeutic process rather than as an 'inadvertent enemy' (p. 104). This is an interesting approach to the treatment of a couple with a depressed partner, given the apparent effectiveness of the cognitive approach for individual therapy. Unfortunately this model has not so far been practised on a wide scale, nor evaluated.

Paykel, Mangen, Griffith and Burns (1982) have conducted a trial in which supportive home visiting by community psychiatric nurses (CPNs) was compared to routine psychiatric out-patient follow-up care for 71 neurotic patients, half of whom had a primary diagnosis of depression. Patients were randomly assigned to either treatment condition and were assessed every 6 months for 18 months. Multiple-outcome criteria were used: symptoms, social functioning, family burden, consumer satisfaction and economic costs were measured. While there were no differences found between the effectiveness of the two treatments on symptoms, social adjustment or family burden, the patients themselves reported greater satisfaction with treatment when they were being visited by CPNs.

From the point of view of supporting families of patients it was not clear that the consumer satisfaction with CPNs extended to relatives. Only about a quarter of patients were found to be in contact with a family with 'a good informant', and thus only 26 per cent of the CPN contacts included the relative. Furthermore the research team reported that perceived family burden tended to be relatively low. They do not elaborate on this finding, and it is not clear why this was the case, given the more general research alluded to earlier on the sorts of problems families typically experience. As this study was primarily designed to look at an alternative professional group's ability to provide an equally good follow-up service to the traditional service, it may not be appropriate to expect that its approach to, and effects on, families would be discussed in detail. Nevertheless, given that this trial did demonstrate that CPNs were able to provide as good a service as out-patient follow-up, and one which patients preferred, the study does suggest that this professional group might well be the ideal one to extend their service and offer more specific support to such families. It would seem likely that relatives might find it easier to accept support in the home setting, and that it might also be effective in offsetting their social isolation.

Finally, my own work offering counselling to the families of long-term schizophrenic and depressed patients and their families is currently being evaluated. Since it has been shown that levels of expressed emotion (EE) in relatives can be changed and relapse rates improved in acute schizophrenic patients and their families (Leff, Kuipers, Berkowitz, Eberlein-Fries and Sturgeon, 1982; Falloon, Boyd, McGill, Razani, Moos and Gilderman, 1982), it may be possible to show some similar effects in a more chronic group. Also, since by the time a mental illness has become established over several years the problems, both for patients and families, have some overlap in different diagnostic groups, it seemed feasible to include depressed as well as schizophrenic patients in the study.

The aim of the intervention is to provide information to relatives in order to improve their understanding and tolerance of symptomatic behaviour, particularly the 'negative symptoms' such as under-

211

activity and social withdrawal, and also to offer long-term support and advice on coping with problems. The education is offered at home using a multiple-choice questionnaire which the relative fills in, and which is discussed in detail afterwards. Things which are misunderstood or answered incorrectly are looked at again and explained by the professional, in this case a psychologist. Relatives are then invited to join a monthly relatives' support group, run by myself and a social worker. During this the relatives are encouraged to talk to each other about common problems and ways of managing. Issues have included medication, the future, diagnosis, independence, guilt, stigma and never having a holiday. It is hoped that as well as providing a forum where relatives may begin to understand some of the problems, and thus have more sympathetic attitudes towards their depressed family members, they may also extend their range of coping responses and reduce their social isolation. This programme is being compared with the more standard care offered to a matched control group, by two other clinical teams in the same building, but results will not be available for at least another year. However it is possible to provide an example of one such family who attend the group irregularly and how they use the facility.

Mr and Mrs Edwards have a 40-year-old son John who has a 17-year history of contact with services. He has been married with four children but the marriage has broken down. After a long period as an in-patient he moved out to his own flat and has survived there for the past year with short admissions to hospital for his frequent manic episodes. However, while ostensibly living alone he visits the parental home several nights a week and at weekends, and his mother cleans his flat and does his laundry at times when he lets this go. The parents are elderly, and the father physically disabled, which restricts their attendance. While very concerned they feel there is little else they can do apart from providing practical support. They are resigned to the fact of his illness but still felt they did not fully understand what it was. This was discussed in some detail in the group, at a time when they were particularly concerned about him, and seemed to help clarify several people's continuing misperception of the illness of their relatives, as well as to reassure them. At the end of the group meetings they said how helpful it had been to share problems, and to know that they were not alone.

Overall, then, while there are suggestions from these studies about the kinds of treatments which might be helpful for families, there is not enough evidence as yet to decide which approach should be preferred. Friedman's marital and drug therapy trial certainly showed promising results for a short-term intervention, but was not followed up and appears not to have been replicated. The cognitive therapy with couples including a depressed partner is innovative but not evaluated. Using CPNs to support families at home has had some success, but has also not been evaluated specifically for this diagnostic group. The information and support group offered in my own study has no results to comment on. Because this study is aimed at a very long-term group of patients, however, it happens that relatives are not typically spouses, marriages often having broken down by this time. Thus the approach here is an alternative one for families where marital therapy would no longer be appropriate. It is possible that the different treatments discussed here actually suit rather different family needs and may well turn out to be complementary. However, the area is undoubtedly in need of some detailed and long-term clinical research on how best to help a range of families with differing problems but all coping with a depressed member.

CONCLUSION

Families living with a depressive disorder are a neglected group who have usually been investigated only as part of the problems experienced by families of all psychiatric patients, and not in their own right. In some ways this is not surprising, as many problems do overlap with those found in families living with other severe psychiatric disorders, particularly if the disorder becomes long-term. However, this neglect has tended to reinforce the attitude that living with a depressed person is in some ways not so difficult. In fact this is not borne out, and the evidence which does exist suggests that the neurotic depressive disorders can be amongst the most difficult to cope with, just because of the overlap with ordinary behaviour patterns and the misinterpretation and tension that can result.

The depressive disorders focus on marriage and relationships because the relative involved is usually a spouse. The devastating effect that such a disorder can have on a relationship, and the changes that can result in both partners — one becoming childlike and dependent, the other having to take over roles and responsibilities while coping with losing their own confidant/e and support — are evident. Children are also likely to be affected, particularly if long-term marital conflict and disruptions accompany the illness. It must not be forgotten, however, that many marriages do survive these problems, and many partners do cope well, and not all spouses exhibit the stresses, strains and neurotic symptoms that are documented for some. It must also be borne in mind that not all relatives are spouses, and that those with the most long-term problems may be living with parents or siblings.

In the search for kinds of help that would be useful clear pointers do exist — relatively straightforward things like information, advice and time off, support and a more positive attitude from professionals involved; some marital help where needed. The availability of this help is virtually non-existent at the present time, and specific help for depressed people and their families has not been a priority. Even self-help groups have hardly got off the ground and there is scope for much more interest and activity in this area.

As was stated initially, depression is not a minor problem and does affect a sizeable number of families. Specialist interest and treatment, as well as self-help groups, focusing on those living and coping with depressive disorders, are long overdue.

REFERENCES

Ambelas, A. (1979) Psychological stressful events in the precipitation of manic episodes, *British Journal of Psychiatry, 135*, 15–21

Bebbington, P.E., Hurry, J. and Tennant, C. (1981) Life events and the nature of psychiatric disorders in the community, *Journal of Affective Disorders, 3*, 345–66

Berkowitz, R., Eberlein-Fries, R., Kuipers, L. and Leff, J. (1984) Educating relatives about schizophrenia, *Schizophrenia Bulletin, 10*, 418–29

Billings, A.G., Cronkite, R.C. and Moos, R.H. (1983) Social-environmental factors in unipolar depression: comparisons of depressed patients and non-depressed patients and non-depressed controls, *Journal of Abnormal Psychology, 92*, 119–33

Birtchnell, J. and Kennard, J. (1983) Does marital maladjustment lead to mental illness? *Social Psychiatry, 18*, 79–88

Brown, G.W. and Harris, T. (1978) *Social origins of depression: a study of psychiatric disorder in women*, Tavistock Publications, London

Brown, G.W., Bhrolchain, M.N. and Harris, T. (1975) Social class and psychiatric disturbance among women in an urban population, *Sociology, 9*, 225–54

Clausen, J.A., Yarrow, M.R., Deasy, L.C. and Schwartz, C.G. (1955) The impact of mental illness: research formulation, *Journal of Social Issues, 11*, 6–11

Collins, J., Kreitman, N., Nelson, B. and Troop, J. (1971) Neurosis and marital interaction. III: Family roles and functions, *British Journal* of Psychiatry, *119*, 233–42

Crammer, L. (1971) Family feedback in depressive illness, *Psychosomatics,* *12*, 127–32

Creer, C., Sturt, E. and Wykes, T. (1982) The role of relatives. In J.K. Wing (ed.), *Long-term community care: experience in a London Borough, Psychological Medicine,* Monograph, Supplement 2, pp. 29–39

Deasy, L.C. and Quinn, O.W. (1955) The wife of the mental patient and the hospital psychiatrist. *Journal of Social Issues, 11*, 49–60

Fadden, G., Bebbington, P. and Kuipers, L. (1987) and its burdens: a study of the relatives of depressed patients, *British Journal of Psychiatry* (in press)

Falloon, I.R.H., Boyd, J.L., McGill, C.W., Razani, J., Moos, H.B. and Gilderman, A.M. (1982) Family management in the prevention of exacerbations of schizophrenia: a controlled study, *New England Journal of Medicine, 306*, 1437–40

Feldman, L.B. (1976) Depression and marital interaction, *Family Process, 15*, 389–95

Friedman, A.S. (1975) Interaction of drug therapy with marital therapy in depressive patients, *Archives of General Psychiatry, 32*, 619–37

Grad, J. and Sainsbury, P. (1963) Mental illness and the family,*Lancet, 1*, 544–7

Hinchliffe, M.K., Hooper, D. and Roberts, F.J. (1978) *The melancholy marriage,* John Wiley and Sons, Chichester.

Hoenig, J. and Hamilton, M.W. (1966) The schizophrenic patient in the community and his effect on the household, *International Journal of Social Psychiatry, 12*, 165–76

Hoenig, J. and Hamilton, M. (1969) *The desegregation of the mentally ill,* Routledge and Kegan Paul, London

Hooley, J.M., Orley, J. and Teasdale, J. (1985) Levels of EE and relapse in depressed patients, *British Journal of Psychiatry, 148*, 642–7

Jacobs,, S.C., Prusoff, B.A. and Paykel E.S. (1974) Recent life events in schizophrenia and depression, *Psychological Medicine, 4*, 444–53

Kennedy, S., Thompson, R., Stancer, H.C., Roy, A. and Persad, E. (1983) Life events precipitating mania, *British Journal of Psychiatry, 142*, 398–403

Kreitman, N. (1964) The patient's spouse, *British Journal of Psychiatry, 110*, 159–73

Kreitman, N., Collins, J., Nelson, B. and Troop, J. (1970) Neurosis and marital interaction. I: Personality and symptoms, *British Journal of Psychiatry, 117*, 33–46

Kuipers, J. and Bebbington, P. (1985) Relatives as a resource in the management of functional illness, *British Journal of Psychiatry, 147*, 465–70

Leff, J.P., Fischer, M. and Bertelsen, A.A. (1976) A cross-national epidemiological study of mania, *British Journal of Psychiatry, 129*, 428–42

Leff, J., Kuipers, L., Berkowitz, R., Eberlein-Fries, R. and Sturgeon, D. (1982) A controlled trial of social intervention in the families of schizophrenic patients, *British Journal of Psychiatry, 141*, 121–34

Lieberman, P.B. and Strauss, J.S. (1984) The recurrence of mania: environmental factors and medical treatment, *American Journal of Psychiatry, 141*, 77–80

Lomas, P. (1967) *The predicament of the family*, Hogarth Press, London

Mann, S. and Cree, W. (1976) 'New' long-stay psychiatric patients: a national sample survey of fifteen mental hospitals in England and Wales 1972/3, *Psychological Medicine, 6*, 603–16

Mills, E. (1962) *Living with mental illness; a study in East London*, Routledge and Kegan Paul, London

Nelson, B., Collins, J., Kreitman, N. and Troop, J. (1970) Neurosis and marital interaction. II: Time sharing and social activity, *British Journal of Psychiatry, 117*, 47–58

Ovenstone, I.M.K. (1973) The development of neurosis in the wives of neurotic men. Part II: Marital role functions and marital tension, *British Journal of Psychiatry, 122*, 711–17

Paykel, E.S. (1978) Contribution of life events to causation of psychiatric illness, *Psychological Medicine, 8*, 245–53

Paykel, E.S. and Tanner, J. (1976) Life events, depressive relapse and maintenance treatment, *Psychological Medicine, 6*, 481–5

Paykel, E.S., Mangen, S., Griffith, J.H. and Burns, T.P. (1982) Community psychiatric nursing for neurotic patients: a controlled trial, *British Journal of Psychiatry, 140*, 573–81

Rush, A.J., Shaw, B. and Khatami, M. (1980) Cognitive therapy of depression: utilising the couples system, *Cognitive Therapy and Research, 4*, 103–13

Rutter, M. (1966) *Children of sick patients: an environmental and psychiatric study*, Maudsley Monograph 16, London University Press, London

Rutter, M. and Quinton, D. (1977) Psychiatric disorder: etiological factors and concepts of causation. In M. McGurk (ed.), *Ecological factors in human development*, North Holland, Amsterdam

Slater, E., Hare, E.H. and Price, J.S. (1971) Marriage and fertility of psychiatric patients compared with national data, *Social Biology, 18*, Supplement, September, 560–73

Sturt, E., Kumakura, N. and Der, G. (1984) How depressing life is — lifelong risk of depressive disorder, a basis for comparison, *Journal of Affective Disorders, 7*, 109–22

Teasdale, J.D. (1985) Non-pharmacological treatments for depression. (Personal communication)

Tuckett, D. (1982) *Final report on the patient project*, Health Education Council, London

Vaughn, C. and Leff, J. (1976) The influence of family and social factors on the course of psychiatric illness. A comparison of schizophrenic and depressed neurotic patients, *British Journal of Psychiatry, 129*, 157–65

Vaughn, C. and Leff, J. (1981) Patterns of relationships, emotional response and family interaction in the families of schizophrenic and depressed patients. (Personal communication)

Weissman, M.S. and Paykel, E.S. (1974) *The depressed woman: a study of social relationships*, University of Chicago Press, Chicago

Yarrow, M.R., Schwartz, C.G., Murphy, H.S. and Deasy, L.C. (1955) The psychological meaning of mental illness in the family, *Journal of Social Issues, 11*, 12–24

10

Chronic Disease in Childhood

Christine Eiser

PSYCHOSOCIAL RAMIFICATIONS OF CHRONIC DISEASE IN CHILDREN

While present-day management of chronic childhood disease is vastly superior to the treatment offered earlier this century, it can also be mechanistic, technological and invasive, and the emotional needs of the patient may well be forgotten in the drive to extend survival. At the turn of this century, children were subject to a number of distressing illnesses, and lack of suitable treatment resulted in premature death for many. Improvements in sanitation, housing and diet, and the introduction of vaccines, have resulted essentially in the eradication of diseases such as polio, tuberculosis and smallpox. At the same time, potentially fatal diseases such as cancer and leukaemia can be treated. The discovery of anti-leukaemia drugs and radiation has improved life-expectancy for children with leukaemia, as have antibiotics for cystic fibrosis. Related improvements in medicine also mean that children who sustain increasingly severe injuries as a result of road accidents or burns can be treated. A rather different story, however, could be told about the psychological impact of such diseases and their treatment on the child and family.

Caring for a chronically sick child is extremely demanding both physically and emotionally. Parents must undertake much of the routine medical care for their child. They must ensure that the child takes required medication. It may be difficult for parents to persuade a child of the need to complete a short course of antibiotics once the symptoms of the illness are passed; it can be extremely difficult in the case of a chronically sick child to ensure co-operation and compliance with instructions over periods of years, and often for life. Many drugs have no immediate effect in alleviating the pain for a chronically sick child. For example, drugs used in the treatment of childhood arthritis have little effect in terms of alleviating acute pain, and can even make the child feel worse. We should not therefore be surprised if the chronically sick child comes to resent the need for drugs and, by implication, those who are responsible for their administration.

The treatment for some chronic diseases is by diet. Some diseases require dramatic changes in the child's diet, and as such are not compatible with the food habits of the rest of the family. Phenylketonuria is a case in point. This inherited disease is the result of a biochemical imbalance and is associated with severe mental subnormality if untreated. The biochemical defect can be corrected by removing all phenylalanine from the child's diet. The treatment must begin within the first few months of life if it is to be successful. Phenylalanine is contained in all protein foods; therefore all meat and dairy products are usually eliminated from the child's diet. Fruit and vegetables are allowed freely. Milk substitutes are available, but the diet remains bland and uninteresting. As children become older they very much resent the lack of variety and restrictions in their diet, and mothers find it difficult to manage. In other cases the child's diet needs to be planned with care, but is not necessarily incompatible with that of the rest of the family. This applies, for example, to the high-roughage diet often recommended for diabetic patients. In addition, many children with asthma are allergic to certain foods. In these cases avoidance of a finite number of foods is usually sufficient to reduce the risk of allergy-induced asthma attacks.

Parents may also need to learn specific tasks to manage their child's illness. Cystic fibrosis may require daily physiotherapy, which can be time-consuming and physically exhausting. Diabetics need to make daily checks of their blood or urine, and adjust their insulin requirements accordingly. Housekeeping can become more complicated; children with asthma may be allergic to house dust. The only solution is to reduce dust by thorough cleaning of the child's room. Other asthmatics may be allergic to animals, and contact must be minimised or eliminated if possible.

The emotional problems for parents are no less daunting. In the first instance, parents must come to terms with the fact that the ambitions they had for the child may never be fulfilled. Illness can compromise achievement by limiting experience and the acquisition of skills or, in the extreme case, by causing premature death. Parents may experience feelings of mourning for the child they hoped to have, feelings not dissimilar from true mourning. While some childhood diseases are relatively stable (for example, juvenile arthritis), others run an unpredictable course. Periods of remission are interspersed by periods of illness. Not knowing if, or when, a crisis may occur can be very difficult to cope with emotionally. Chronic disease is usually defined as a condition which lasts for more than 3 months and for which no cure is available. Parents naturally nurture the hope that a miracle drug will be discovered. For some children there is a reasonable hope that the severity of the disease will lessen as the child grows. This is especially true for asthma, although the myth that children routinely 'outgrow' asthma at 7 years is largely unfounded. Many children never outgrow the condition. In other diseases there is little hope that the child will do anything but remain stable, or even deteriorate, over the years. Increasingly parents also worry about long-term complications of the disease. Diabetes, for example, is associated with risk to the vascular, retinal and neural systems. For the diabetic, blindness is particularly difficult. The inability to conduct one's own urine and blood tests and manage injections may increase personal feelings of dependence and inadequacy. It is unfortunately also true that the risk of serious complications increases with the length of survival. Thus the younger the child on diagnosis the greater the risk of development of complications. There are anxieties, too, about complications and dependence developing from long-term use of necessary drugs. Parents of children with asthma and epilepsy are probably the most concerned. In addition, children with chronic disease often seem especially prone to other, minor complaints. Ordinary coughs and colds can precipitate asthma attacks for some children. Those with leukaemia can develop fatal complications following ordinary childhood complaints, especially measles.

Child-rearing can be an exhausting business at any time, but the difficulties are exacerbated in the case of chronic disease. Nights may be disrupted as a result of the disease, or because of pain and sickness associated with the treatment. Not surprisingly, anxiety and exhaustion take their toll, and family life is disrupted. Parents have little time or energy left for each other, and little opportunity to discuss their anxieties without also distressing other children. A higher incidence of family discord, marital separation and divorce, increased psychiatric complaints among parents, especially mothers, and emotional and behavioural disturbance among healthy siblings have all been linked to chronic childhood disease.

Yet this view needs to be seen in perspective. While nobody could deny the enormous burden that is associated with rearing a sick child, there appear to be compensations. It is very unusual for parents to express regret that treatment was undertaken, even in situations where the disease proves fatal. Increasingly there are reports that families are drawn closer together as a result of caring for the child; they see each other and their ambitions in a new light. The children who survive chronic disease are not left unscathed by the experience. The misery of the disease and awareness of pain experienced may recede, but their lives are irreversibly changed. Anecdotal reports suggest that the survivors of chronic disease often show unusual degrees of empathy and sympathy with others, and choose caring or nursing professions.

There have been three large epidemiological surveys concerned with the incidence of disease in the child population. In the 'National Survey' (Pless and Douglas, 1971), 5300 children resident in the United Kingdom were followed longitudinally. The 'Rochester' sample (Pless and Roghmann, 1971) included a 1 per cent sample (N = 1756) of children under 18 years living in Monroe County, New York, and the 'Isle of Wight' survey (Rutter, Graham and Yule, 1970) included the total resident population of 9-11-year-old children. Estimates of the incidence of chronic childhood disease were similar in all three studies (10–12 per cent). Mattson (1972) later reported that the most common illnesses included asthma (2 per cent), epilepsy (1 per cent), cardiac conditions (0.5 per cent), cerebral palsy (0.5 per cent), orthopaedic illnesses (0.5 per cent) and diabetes mellitus (0.1 per cent). There is other evidence that the incidence of diabetes is increasing, and several studies point to the incidence of asthma being more than 2 per cent.

Recognition of the relatively high numbers of children affected by chronic disease, and the increasingly technological nature of much treatment, has led to a mushrooming of research into the psychological repercussions for child and family. There is an increasing awareness that success in paediatric medicine cannot, and should not, be measured in terms of survival alone. It is essential also that the child's 'quality of life' is not unnecessarily compromised. It is generally agreed that paediatric medicine should have at least three aims:

1. to treat the disease itself,
2. to prevent the disease from interfering with the *child's development*, and
3. to prevent the disease from adversely affecting the *family*.

Most psychological research falls neatly into sections 2 or 3. For the most part there is little acknowledgement of the fact that the course of the child's development is determined not only by the disease, but also by the reactions and support offered by the family. Conversely, the family's reaction is determined in part by how successfully the child comes to terms with the disease and its management; in part by whether complications set in and the child's health deteriorates more than expected. For instance, Mattson (1972) reported that children who were poorly adjusted to their disease had parents who were (1) fearful and protective, (2) oversolicitous and guilt-ridden or (3) embarrassed and ashamed. Jay, Ozolins, Elliot and Caldwell (1983) examined the behaviour of children with leukaemia undergoing extremely painful bone marrow aspirations (BMA); a routine part of leukaemia treatment and essential in order to enable early diagnosis of relapse. Children under 7 years of age showed much greater stress than older children, but, in addition, children whose parents scored higher on anxiety scales showed significantly more stress than the children of parents with lower scores. Of course, it is very distressing for parents to have to watch their child undergo these procedures, and it may be that if a child reacts in a very overt, distressed way the parents would become especially anxious. An alternative explanation might be that parents who were anxious generally about hospitals and treatment were likely to communicate these attitudes to the child, and thus increase the child's levels of stress. The 'chicken-and-egg' nature of this problem has deterred many investigators, but this does not mean that we should forget how closely related are the attitudes and behaviour of child and family. In the remainder of this chapter, however, the two will be considered separately, since most research falls primarily under one or other heading.

IMPACT OF CHRONIC DISEASE ON THE CHILD

This section is a brief and selective review of the literature, since the focus of this book is on *family* reactions to stress. The question that long-term chronic illness might compromise normal child development is, however, a real one, and in itself likely to affect family functioning. It is one thing for family members to come to terms with chronic illness and the demands of treatment; it is quite another for them to contend also with slow intellectual development or deviant behaviour. There is some evidence that chronic illness brings an increased risk of abnormal development in both these contexts.

Of particular concern has been the issue of whether intelligence in the chronically sick child is adversely affected. There are many

221

reasons for expecting that it might be. The illness may limit the child's opportunity to experience or manipulate the environment, and this lack of opportunity may result in reduced intellectual functioning. Parents may be overprotective and limit the child's activities unnecessarily. Markova, Stirling-Phillips and Forbes (1984) found that parents of boys with haemophilia, so as to reduce the possibility of injury, provided little opportunity for the children to handle sharp tools. The result was that the boys were unskilled with tools. Consequently they were careless and more likely to have an accident than healthy boys who had learned how to use such tools with care. Parents and teachers may expect very little of the sick child, feeling that the child should be able to enjoy life if possible without being subject to the same discipline as other children. Either because of the illness, or associated minor complaints and hospital visits, the sick child often has a poorer school attendance record.

In fact, most research suggests that children with chronic disease have IQ scores within the normal range, but their school achievements (as measured largely by tests of reading) lag considerably behind those of healthy children. These findings raise questions about how children with chronic disease are treated in normal schools. Many parents and medical staff see the attendance at normal school as essential for sick children, in all but the most exceptional circumstances. Attendance at normal school enables the sick child to mix with children of similar age as well as live at home. (Distance from home often means that the sick child attending special school has to live away from home, isolating the child from the family and reducing the likelihood of forming close friendships with local children.) Many parents, too, often prefer the child to go to a local school, largely because they see the education as better or want the child to be treated as normally as possible. In fact the 1981 Education Act states that all sick or handicapped children have the right to be taught in normal schools. Teachers themselves, however, sometimes have reservations about accepting children into their class whom they perceive as potentially difficult to teach and frequently absent. In addition, teachers can be very apprehensive about teaching children with conditions such as asthma or epilepsy, since they anticipate difficulties in handling episodes of illness if they occur in the class. Certainly teachers have very little training in teaching such children, and appear inadequately informed about childhood disease.

For chronically sick children and their families, the return to school following diagnosis is a major event. It signifies the end of the immediate crisis and continuity with a style of life more similar to the rest of the population. For the mother, it coincides with a freedom from the constant presence of the sick child and the burden of being both nurse and mother. However, there has been a rather naive assumption on the part of medical personnel that the transition back to school will be plain sailing. We know now that this is not always so.

IMPACT OF CHRONIC DISEASE ON THE FAMILY

We should not be surprised to find that much research has pointed out the adverse repercussions of chronic childhood illness for the parents' mental health, their relationship with each other, their relationship with the sick child, and communication within the family generally. Healthy siblings, too, are reported to show adverse behavioural and emotional reactions (for a general review, see Eiser, 1985).

Increasingly there is also evidence that some families cope effectively with the demands of treatment and enforced changes in style of life. Some authors go so far as to suggest that there can be real positive benefits to the family in terms of increased understanding, empathy and greater depths of feeling towards each other. The literature concerned with the effects of chronic childhood illness and divorce rates illustrates these extreme views well. Early findings consistently reported that childhood illness was associated with increased divorce rates. In contrast, Schulman (1976) reported that caring for a child with leukaemia had the effect of drawing families together. These results are often reconciled by suggesting that the occurrence of chronic illness accentuates the strengths and weaknesses of pre-existing relationships. Thus, in weak marriages, the child's illness increases tension; in 'good' marriages the illness further cements relationships.

Much work has looked at families' reactions to chronic illness at diagnosis. Other work has focused on attitudes at the time of the child's death and parents' recovery from mourning. Far less attention has been paid to how families cope with day-to-day demands either of a practical or emotional nature during the course of the illness.

Reactions at diagnosis

Parents' reactions to the diagnosis of a chronic or life-threatening disease in their child is first reported to be one of *shock* or *disbelief*. This phase is followed by a longer period of *denial*, in which parents may seek alternative opinions about the child's health. At the same time, parents report intense feelings of anger and frustration. Anger may be directed by parents at each other, or at medical staff, or God. Parents may feel that medical staff are not doing enough for their child, or failed to diagnose the condition early enough. They also often exert considerable effort towards learning and understanding about the disease, a process sometimes described as *intellectualisation*. Parents also may experience extreme guilt feelings, questioning if they sought medical advice early enough, or if they precipitated the disease by some action of their own. Mothers particularly may worry that they drank or smoked too much during pregnancy. Of longest duration is the *adaptive* phase, during which child and family learn to manage the illness and its demands with as little intrusion into other activities as possible.

Moos and Tsu (1977) see adaptation to illness as the acquisition of a series of skills. Skills are first acquired which are aimed at minimising the seriousness of the disease. This is followed by attempts to seek information and learn about the disease. Thirdly, individuals lobby emotional support and reassurance from family, friends and professionals. Fourthly, individuals learn specific illness-related procedures (including, for example, how to give insulin injections for the diabetic, or specific allergens to be avoided in the case of the asthmatic). Fifthly, realistic goals must be set up and difficult tasks broken down into manageable parts. During the acquisition of the sixth skill the patient must develop strategies appropriate for coping with everyday aspects of life. In the final stage the patients' ambitions and hopes need to be put in perspective, and new realistic goals identified.

Longitudinal studies

Few would expect anything other than the reactions of intense grief and shock generally observed in parents to the diagnosis of a chronically sick child. For this reason, parents can expect considerable support and help. Neighbours and relations are at first very willing to mind other children, give lifts to the hospital or cook meals. Medical and paramedical staff are prepared to discuss the diagnosis and its implications at considerable length. It is after the initial stage that parents can feel let down. Once the child is out of hospital there is less help from medical staff, less opportunity to discuss the illness with staff or other parents, while at the same time parents take on full-time responsibility for the medical care of their child. Neighbours and friends progressively reduce the amount of help offered, and may slowly withdraw all contact as they regard the situation as increasingly hopeless and depressing. Parents may also feel quite unprepared to tackle many of the problems involved, and feel very insecure and anxious in the absence of medical staff to turn to for advice. Quite unexpected difficulties can be encountered. For example, the child's return to school can be traumatic with peers and teachers feeling hesitant and appearing hostile. In addition, the course of many chronic diseases is unpredictable. While some children may appear relatively fit and slot back into their old routines with little problem, other children can experience considerable ill-health and setbacks. For all these reasons the longitudinal study of families coping with chronic disease is essential, if professional help can be made available as necessary. Unfortunately there have been fewer of these studies than might have been hoped. Research that has been published tends to be limited to more 'dramatic' diseases, especially cancer and leukaemia, while we know little in this context about children with asthma and their families. Such an omission needs correction in the near future.

Several longitudinal studies of families coping with leukaemia and cancer can be cited. Maguire, Comaroff, Ramsell and Morris-Jones (1979) interviewed the parents of 60 children with leukaemia over a period of 12–18 months. Their responses were compared with a group of parents whose children suffered from benign disease. Maguire *et al.* found a high incidence of problems for the families of leukaemia children immediately following diagnosis and at follow-up. In the period following diagnosis, 30 per cent of mothers of leukaemia children were considered to be highly anxious. They reported being on edge, unable to relax or sleep well and couldn't stop thinking about the child's illness. Similar feelings were reported by only 5 per cent of mothers of children with benign disease. Over one-third of mothers of leukaemia children and 9 per cent of mothers of children with benign disease showed symptoms of depression. At follow-up, one-quarter of the mothers of leukaemia children were still highly anxious or depressed, compared with 8 per cent of mothers of children with benign disease. In their conclusions, Maguire *et al.* state that a substantial proportion of mothers of children with leukaemia develop psychiatric problems. While most are mild or moderate in severity, the adverse reactions continue at least for the first 18 months following diagnosis.

A similar study was conducted by Kupst, Schulman, Honig, Maurer, Morgan and Fochtman (1982). These authors studied the families of 64 children with leukaemia from diagnosis until 12 months later. Over the 1-year period there were significant fluctuations in the family's reported responses to the disease. In contradistinction to the Maguire study, the overall picture that emerges from the work of Kupst *et al.* is relatively optimistic. They interpret their data as indicating that the majority of families cope well with the disease 1 year post-diagnosis. (In fact, only 15 of the 64 families were rated as coping poorly at 1 year.) Kupst *et al.* argue that the families who cope poorly are those who have pre-existing problems, a view which is beginning to emerge with some consistency (Schulman and Kupst, 1980).

Sixty of the children and their families were followed up again 2 years after diagnosis (Kupst, Schulman, Maurer, Honig, Morgan and Fochtman, 1984). (At this time, 44 (73.3 per cent) of the children remained well and in remission.) Families of children in remission were reported to be coping well 2 years after diagnosis. This statement was based both on ratings made of the families by medical staff and on the fact that families scored within the normal range on standardised measures of family coping. Measures of coping at diagnosis, 1 year and 2 years post-diagnosis were significantly related. Kupst *et al.* (1984) point out that while most families appeared to be coping well, the ways in which they coped were diverse.

> Coping with pediatric leukaemia took many forms. Some people focused on problems connected with the illness, while others minimized the severity of the crisis. Some freely showed their feelings of anxiety, apprehension, sadness, or anger, while others maintained a cheerful or positive attitude. A number of family members relied on religion or faith, but many did not. While open communication and an attitude of living in the present correlated with coping, the influence of other modes and strategies was unclear. (Kupst *et al.*, 1984, pp. 160–1)

The apparent discrepancies between the studies reported by Maguire *et al.* (1979) and those by Kupst *et al.* (1982, 1984) might be attributed to several factors. The first is cultural. Maguire *et al.* worked in England; Kupst *et al.* in the United States. Subtle differences in terms of treatment of the disease may be important, but so also may be cultural differences in the perceptions of severe illness. While Maguire *et al.* (1979) reported that all children with leukaemia diagnosed within a given period were followed up, Kupst *et al.* (1982) acknowledged that a proportion of their families were not able to be contacted at 1 year post-diagnosis. Some did not want to participate, whether because they were too depressed to be involved or, as Kupst *et al.* (1982) speculate, were sufficiently well-adapted to the disease that they did not wish to be reminded is open to question. Sample attrition is always a problem in interpreting data of this kind.

A third problem relates to the type of questions and interview schedules that were used to assess families. Research of this kind too often assumes that chronic illness will have a devastating impact on children and their families, and interview schedules are then designed to investigate these negative effects. In this way any positive effects of the disease in terms of bringing families closer together, or increasing empathy with others, is not investigated. Some differences between the two studies can therefore be attributed to differences in emphasis adopted by the two sets of researchers. Taken together, however, both studies point to a decrease in psychiatric symptoms among families during the 12 months following diagnosis. The work by Kupst *et al.* (1982) goes a little way in describing which families are most likely to show adverse reactions to the disease. Families coped particularly poorly who expressed high levels of stress in addition to stresses associated with the disease. In particular, the experience of financial difficulties and pregnancy increased the likelihood that a family was seen as not coping well with the disease. Kupst *et al.* (1984) also point to the different ways in which coping has been conceptualised. Anger, for example, may be viewed as part of a normal adaptation process (Futterman and Hoffman, 1973) or as a pathological indicator. Similarly, denial is perceived by some researchers to serve an adaptive function, by others as indicative of maladjustment. Conclusions about how well families cope with chronic illness are therefore in part determined by the definition of coping adopted.

Other work of a longitudinal nature has centred on families' reactions to diabetes. In the now classic study, Koski (1969) divided 60 children with diabetes into two groups on the basis of their metabolic control. (Some children have what is sometimes called a 'brittle' form of the disease, with frequent episodes of hypoglycaemia resulting in hospitalisation.) Koski reported that the initial reactions of grief and shock described earlier were followed within a few weeks by reasonable adjustment. Mothers of children in good control were more expressive and emotional in their original reactions, and mothers of those in poor control tended to be less expressive and denied their emotions. In follow-up 5 years later, Koski and Kumento (1975) reported that nine patients who had originally been classified as in poor control had changed to good control. Some children who were originally in good control had changed to poor control, but all of these came from families characterised by high degrees of stress and disruption. Finally, Kovacs (1981) was interested specifically in the effects of the diagnosis of childhood diabetes on parents. Kovacs reported that, for marriages with no history of marital problems, no problems were identified 1 year following diagnosis. However, families where there was a history of marital problems continued to experience difficulties.

In all research of this type it is remarkable how resilient families can be despite the inordinate stress that the diagnosis and management of chronic childhood disease can bring. The findings regarding parents' reactions to the death of their child follow a very similar pattern.

Reactions to death

For the child with chronic disease parents may begin the mourning process on diagnosis. For those suffering from cancer or leukaemia it may well be that the disease does not prove fatal for several years after the diagnosis. In these cases, parents experience 'anticipatory mourning'. The process is thought to be adaptive, allowing parents to grieve in a slower, more adaptive manner. This avoids the intense grief experienced when a child is stillborn or born with a congenital defect, where no opportunity for anticipatory mourning can occur.

Early studies were largely descriptive and confined to the period immediately following the child's death. More recent work has focused on identifying those variables which might predict how well a family will recover following the child's death. In this respect the study by Rando (1983) is one of the most comprehensive. Rando studied mothers and fathers of 27 children who died, for 3 years after the child's death. She questions previously accepted findings that grief reactions lessen over time, and noted that for many parents, grief intensified over the 3-year period. She also questioned previous findings that mothers are more adversely affected by a child's death than fathers; both parents exhibiting similar patterns of grief and adjustment. Parents whose child had been ill for more than 18 months, and who had experienced previous loss, were the most poorly adjusted.

IMPLICATIONS OF RESEARCH FOR PRACTICE

One of the principal aims of much of the research cited is in the implications for improved medical and psychological services to children and their families. It is also the basis on which many families agree to participate in research, which for them can be emotionally painful and traumatic. This is especially true, for example, of research in which parents are asked about their reactions to the death of a child. While a proportion of families may benefit from being given the opportunity to discuss events and experiences of such a painful nature, others will always find such involvement too harrowing, and decline to participate. The extent to which individual families benefit personally from participating in research may be limited. In this final section the aim is to look at how far research has implications for the care of future patients, and whether any changes in policy are called for.

I argued at the beginning of this chapter that the responses of children and their families to chronic illness are intimately related; the child who copes well tends to come from a family that copes well, and vice versa. Therefore it might be expected that interventions aimed at the child might have positive repercussions for both child and family. Other interventions, aimed primarily at the family, could nevertheless be expected to influence the child. In this final section interventions aimed primarily at the child and family are discussed separately, but their implications for each other should not be overlooked.

INTERVENTIONS WITH THE CHRONICALLY SICK CHILD

Interventions range from broad-based educational techniques aimed at improving knowledge of the disease and self-care behaviours among children, to more intense clinical programmes designed to overcome specific problems as they occur for individuals. Educational techniques have largely centred on offering help to children with asthma or diabetes. In an attempt to improve self-care behaviour of children with asthma, Lewis, Rachelefsky, Lewis, de la Suta and Kaplan (1984) assigned 76 children to either a control or experimental group. The control group received 4½ hours of lectures on asthma management. The experimental group received five 1-hour sessions designed to show the extent to which children with asthma had a degree of control over their disease. The theme of the sessions revolved round likening asthma to driving a car, and the child was taught how to control the disease by avoiding allergens and irritants, to control asthma by using drugs, and how to develop relaxation skills and breathing exercises. Both groups subsequently showed an increase in disease-related knowledge. However, children in the experimental group also reported an increase in compliance behaviour and reduction in number of days of emergency hospitalisation. Of special interest is the fact that Lewis *et al.* claimed that these changes were mediated through improvements in family dynamics. Parents of children in the experimental group were more likely to report improvements in family communication. They also reported reducing the frequency with which they smoked in front of the children (cigarette smoke can exacerbate episodes of respiratory distress for children with asthma). Thus, even though intervention was aimed at the child rather than the whole family, the effect was such that improvements were noted not only in the child's behaviour but also for communication and behaviour within the family as a whole.

Most research of this kind has, however, been conducted with children with diabetes. For young children, and those newly diagnosed, it is clear that parents assume virtually all responsibility for the daily tests and injections needed to control the disease. Yet self-care is considered very important for these children, and much research has focused on when children can successfully assume responsibility for their own tests and injections. Recent research suggests that in the past children may have been encouraged to be more independent about self-care than was optimal, since their ability to handle practical aspects of self-care is dependent on their cognitive maturity. This implies that children with diabetes are unable to handle certain information or translate it into practical terms, below a specified age. This was demonstrated particularly in a study by Harkavy, Johnson, Silverstein, Spillar, McCallum and Rosenbloom (1983). In this study children with diabetes attended summer camp, and their knowledge of the disease and skill in interpreting tests and giving injections was assessed at the beginning and end of the camp. Children aged between 12 and 15 years showed significant improvement in both knowledge and skill over the two occasions. A group of 10-year-olds showed no improvement at all. It is concluded that adolescents are able to benefit from teaching about diabetes, but younger children lack the sufficient cognitive skills for similar benefits to accrue. The data may suggest that some family disagreements could be avoided if parents were more patient about when their children could be entirely self-sufficient with regard to the disease.

There exists a range of techniques of a more therapeutic kind aimed at specific problems experienced by children and their families. Perhaps one of the most popular is *play therapy*. The programme of activities included in play therapy may vary from simple recreation to a continuum of activities derived from theoretical principles. A broadly based definition of play therapy requires: (1) the participation of a professional worker, (2) the use of play to express fear or conflict and master anxiety and (3) the use of identifiable therapeutic goals. Play therapy has been associated with a degree of success in individual case studies. Oremland and Oremland (1973) treated a 5-year-old with malignancy, and using tinker toys and stuffed animals, claimed that the child was able to overcome fear of medical machinery. Plank and Horwood (1977) reported on a 4-year-old girl who underwent surgery for a leg amputation and was helped in rehabilitation by playing with a similar doll. One of the difficulties in using play therapy relates to how questions raised by children during the play sessions are to be answered. The programme needs to be worked out carefully so that the child's questions can be answered honestly without raising additional fears. Conventional play therapy may also be used successfully with children of poor verbal ability, although McDonnell (1979) achieved some success by using art work to aid communication with the less verbal child.

Group play therapy has also been associated with some success. Hoffman and Futterman (1971) devised a programme of group play and activities for use in the waiting room of an oncology clinic. These clinics can be extremely stressful for children, families and patients. Children usually attend very frequently (on average once every 3 weeks). Families are anxious since they must wait several hours for the results of tests which indicate if the child remains well and in 'remission', or if 'relapse' has occurred and treatment needs to be intensified. Children who do relapse show a much-reduced probability of survival. Since families attend these clinics for many years, they become quite friendly with each other. While this serves some positive functions in enabling families to talk and get to know others in a similar position, the disadvantage is that a setback suffered by one child is apparent and stressful to the rest of the clinic. A child who dies is noticeably absent from the regular clinic, and this heightens the tension experienced by other families and staff. Claims made by Hoffman and Futterman (1971) that group play therapy led to an improved atmosphere in such a clinic therefore has important implications, both for the treatment of oncology patients and the potential value of play therapy. A related study by Irwin and McWilliams (1974) involved pre-schoolers with cleft lip or palate in a year-long programme of

231

group play therapy focusing on drama activities. At the end of the year there were significant improvements in speech and behaviour. Play therapy has also been used successfully to prepare children for painful or traumatic surgery (Schwartz, Albino and Tedesco, 1983).

INTERVENTIONS WITH THE FAMILY

One of the simplest interventions used with families involves the provision of a support system. This may involve a professional working with individuals or groups, or may depend more on providing a network of contacts so that families in similar situations can support each other. One of the first reports of this kind was made by Pless and Satterwhite (1972). They trained six women (four of whom had a child with chronic disease) to serve as counsellors. Between them the women worked with 48 families, making home visits as well as offering advice and information by telephone. For the most part, mothers appeared happy with the service, and subsequently rated their children as better adjusted psychologically than a control group of mothers who received no support.

Probably the best-known type of support group is Alcoholics Anonymous, but many other groups have sprung up in recent years designed to help people manage specific obsessive or compulsive behaviours. Virtually wherever you live, it is possible to join a group of people working together to lose weight, drink or smoke less. The aims behind all support groups are to provide: (1) the awareness that the individual is not alone with the problem, (2) awareness of a variety of solutions to handle the problem, (3) models who have overcome or are tackling the problem successfully, and (4) help in coping with the stigma of the obsession or compulsion or disease.

Attempts to set up similar support groups for sick children and their families have been described. These may vary as to whether or not medical personnel are included. Groups may consist of parents only, children only, or parents and children. Some workers offer a finite number of sessions; others let the group run its course. In addition, the programme of discussion can vary from specific topics thought to be of general concern, to more general issues. The assumption that underlies this approach is that interaction with families facing similar crises can be therapeutic. By discussing personal experiences, recognising that these are not unique, and becoming aware of how others tackle similar problems, it is hoped that families will derive some mutual benefit. The ideals behind this approach are often highly commendable; however there is very little research directed at the question of how successful the groups really are in their aims.

An alternative, but equally popular, intervention involves *family therapy*. Lask (1985) describes family therapy as

> a way of conceptualising how problems may be perpetuated, and in some cases initiated, by the family. Childhood problems, be they behavioural or physical, can play an essential part in maintaining family stability, while the family's particular way of handling them may perpetuate the symptoms. (Lask, 1985, p. 297)

Advocates of family therapy see no advantage in using individually orientated therapy, since this would not address the real problem within the family relationships. Family therapy is thought to be particularly promising in dealing with childhood illness where a psychological component may well be involved in causing or aggravating the condition (for example asthma or diabetes), as well as in other chronic childhood conditions which may have adverse consequences for the family (for example renal disease or cystic fibrosis).

The first stage of the intervention involves assessment of family functioning. This includes three components: taking a family history, asking for details of the problem and an examination. In the examination the family are observed together. Observations are made of what is said between family members, the closeness or distance between individuals, how the family communicates and how emotions are expressed. On this basis the therapist may make recommendations about what appear to be the main problems for the family. In chronic illness it is particularly common for the mother and child to become so close that other family relationships are jeopardised, and the therapist would attempt to help mother and child accept a greater degree of independence from each other. Much success has been claimed in treating families of children with conditions such as asthma or diabetes with family therapy.

CONCLUSIONS AND RECOMMENDATIONS FOR HELPING CHRONICALLY SICK CHILDREN AND THEIR FAMILIES

Improvements in the medical care of children with chronic diseases has been impressive in recent years; the need for similar high-quality psychological care is only now being recognised. There is no doubt that the occurrence of such a disease in a child increases the risk to normal child development, parental mental health and family relationships. The fact that some children and their families appear to manage well should not allow us to be complacent about the quality or quantity of care available.

Sick children need help in understanding the cause of the disease and reasons for treatment. These children can be very confused about details of the disease process and its implications. Some young children believe that disease is a punishment, or the result of a magic spell. Young children with diabetes, for example, may think that their illness is a punishment for eating too much sugar. Beliefs such as these may well colour the child's attitude to treatment, and behaviour towards medical personnel, and should be carefully considered. More research effort could be directed at unravelling children's beliefs about illness so that we are able to understand their confusions.

Sick children also need considerable help on return to school. There is the obvious need to provide remedial help to overcome the adverse effects of school absence. Less obvious is the need to help children establish friendships and status among peers. Low Guat Tin and Teasdale (1985) report that children with spina bifida attending normal school spend less time in interactions with others than healthy classmates. Peers were less likely to initiate interaction with the spina bifida children, perhaps signifying their low acceptability. It is likely that all chronically sick children will need help with peer relationships. The attitudes and behaviour of healthy children to the chronically sick are likely to be strongly influenced by the behaviour of their teachers. For this reason, teachers must be made aware of their important role. Education must be aimed at teachers to ensure that they welcome sick children back to school, and foster good relationships among the children.

It is devastating for parents to learn that their child has a chronic condition, but there has been some progress in the extent to which support and help is available. Most paediatric wards do encourage parents (or mothers at least) to stay in hospital with their child. In the most recent survey of hospital practice, Thornes (1983) found that 89 per cent of wards in which children were nursed were in a position to offer overnight accommodation to parents. They are encouraged to be responsible for everyday care of their child, such as feeding, bathing and changing where necessary, while at the same time parents can learn some of the more specialist skills necessary to cope with the disease. This in itself means that parents and children are not separated during diagnosis or subsequent hospitalisation. Parental need for information is also being increasingly recognised. Staff on paediatric units are generally more concerned to answer questions than those on adult wards. Support groups are often set up in the hospital, and there are also many local branches of self-help societies. Most help tends to be directed at the mother. In the future there needs to be greater recognition of the fact that chronic childhood disease is a diagnosis that affects the whole family. The attitude of the father is vital. The disease also has repercussions for healthy siblings. These children tend to view their parents as over-indulgent towards the sick child. They may also feel isolated and deprived, and excluded from the rest of the family. Reactions may be particularly extreme following a sibling's death. Parents do often exclude healthy siblings from discussions of the illness and visits to the hospital, under the usually misguided belief that this will lessen the child's anxiety. Parents need to be made aware that their healthy children have needs too, and involve them in the care of the sick child as far as possible.

REFERENCES

Eiser, C. (1985) *The psychology of childhood illness*, Springer-Verlag, New York

Futterman, E. H. and Hoffman, I. (1973) Crisis and adaptation in families of fatally ill children. In E.J. Anthony and C. Koupernick (eds), *The child in his family: the impact of disease and death*, Wiley, New York, pp. 127–43

Harkavy, J., Johnson, S.B., Silverstein, J., Spillar, R., McCallum, M. and Rosenbloom, A. (1983) Who learns what at diabetes summer camp? *Journal of Pediatric Psychology, 8*, 143–53

Hoffman, I. and Futterman, E.H. (1971) Coping with waiting: psychiatric intervention and study in the waiting room of a pediatric oncology clinic, *Comprehensive Psychiatry, 12*, 67–81

Irwin, E.C. and McWilliams, B.J. (1974) Play therapy for children with cleft palates, *Children Today, 3*, 18–22

Jay, S.M., Ozolins, M., Elliot, C.H. and Caldwell, S. (1983) Assessment of children's distress during painful medical procedures, *Health Psychology, 2*, 133–47

Koski, M.L. (1969) The coping processes in childhood diabetes, *Acta Paediatrica Scandinavia, 198* (Suppl.), 7–56

Koski, M.L. and Kumento, A. (1975) Adolescent development and behaviour: a psychosomatic follow-up of childhood diabetes. In Z. Laron (ed.), *Modern problems in paediatrics*, Vol. 12: *Diabetes in juveniles: medical and rehabilitation aspects*, Karger, Basel, pp. 348–53

Kovacs, M. (1981) The psychosocial sequelae of the diagnosis of juvenile diabetes on the parents of the youngsters. Paper presented at the 5th International Beilinson Symposium on Psychosocial Aspects of Diabetes in Children and Adolescents, Herzliya-on-See, Israel

Kupst, M.J., Schulman, J.L., Honig, G., Maurer, H., Morgan, E. and Fochtman, D. (1982) Family coping with childhood leukaemia: one year after diagnosis, *Journal of Pediatric Psychology, 7*, 157–74

Kupst, M.J., Schulman, J.L., Maurer, H., Honig, G., Morgan, E. and Fochtman, D. (1984) Coping with pediatric leukaemia: a two-year follow-up, *Journal of Pediatric Psychology, 9*, 149–64

Lask, B. (1985) Family therapy, *Archives of Disease in Childhood, 60*, 297–8

Lewis, C.E., Rachelefsky, G., Lewis, M.A., de la Suta, A. and Kaplan, M. (1984). A randomized trial of A.C.T. (asthma care training) for kids, *Pediatrics, 74*, 478–86

Low Guat Tin and Teasdale, G.R. (1985) An observational study of the social adjustment of spina bifida children in integrated settings, *British Journal of Educational Psychology, 55*, 81–3

McDonnell, L. (1979) Paraverbal therapy in pediatric cases with emotional complications, *American Journal of Orthopsychiatry, 49*, 44–52

Maguire, P., Comaroff, J., Ramsell, P.L. and Morris-Jones, P.H. (1979) Psychological and social problems in families of children with leukaemia. In P.H. Morris-Jones (ed.), *Topics in paediatrics*, Vol. 1: *Haematology and oncology*, Pitman Medical, London, pp. 141–9

Markova, I., Stirling-Phillips, J. and Forbes, C.D. (1984) The use of tools by children with haemophilia, *Journal of Child Psychology and Psychiatry, 25*, 261–72

Mattson, A. (1972) Long-term physical illness in childhood: a challenge to psychosocial adaptation, *Pediatrics, 50*, 801–11

Moos, R.H. and Tsu, V.D. (1977) The crisis of physical illness: an overview. In R.H. Moos (ed.), *Coping with physical illness*, Plenum, New York

Oremland, E.K. and Oremland, J.D. (eds) (1973) *The effects of hospitalization on children: models for their care*, Charles C. Thomas, Springfield, Illinois

Plank, E.N. and Horwood, C. (1977) Leg amputation in a four year old: reactions of the child, her family and the staff. In *An anthology of the psychoanalytic study of the child: physical illness and handicap in childhood*, Yale University Press, New Haven

Pless, I.B. and Douglas, J.W.B. (1971) Chronic illness in childhood. 1: Epidemiological and clinical characteristics, *Pediatrics, 47*, 405–14

Pless, I.B. and Pinkerton, P. (1975) *Chronic childhood disorder promoting patterns of adjustment*, Henry Kimpton, London

Pless, I.B. and Roghmann, K.J (1971) Chronic illness and its consequences: observations based on three epidemiological surveys, *Journal of Pediatrics, 79*, 351–9

Pless, I.B. and Satterwhite, B. (1972) Chronic illness in childhood: selection, activities and evaluation of non-professional family counselors, *Clinical Pediatrics, 11*, 403–10

Rando, T.A. (1983) An investigation of grief and adaptation in parents whose children have died from cancer, *Journal of Pediatric Psychology, 8*, 3–20

Rutter, M., Graham, P. and Yule, W. (1970) *A neuropsychiatric study in childhood*. Clinics in Developmental Medicine, No. 35/36, SIMP/ Heinemann, London

Schulman, J.L. (1976) *Coping with tragedy: successfully facing the problem of a seriously ill child*, Follett, Chicago, Illinois

Schulman J.L. and Kupst, M.J. (eds) (1980) *The child with cancer. Clinical approaches to psychological care: research in psychosocial aspects*, C.C. Thomas, Springfield, Illinois

Schwartz, D.D.S., Albino, J.E. and Tedesco, L. (1983) Effects of psychological preparation on children hospitalized for dental operations, *Journal of Pediatrics, 102*, 634–8

Thornes, R. (1983) Parental access and family facilities in children's wards in England, *British Medical Journal, 287*, 190–2

11

Brain Damage and the Family

Nick Moffat

In this chapter the problems that may be of concern to the family and the person who has acquired brain damage are discussed, including the initial shock of learning that a person has brain damage, the feelings of loss, the processes of adjustment to the problems, and the readjustment following improvements, or possibly the death of the affected person. In addition, general ways of coping are described, together with particular strategies for coping with the more typical problems after brain damage, such as impaired memory. The final section explores various ways in which professionals may help the family to cope.

TYPES OF BRAIN DAMAGE

An overview is provided of the types of problems experienced by families who have a member with acquired brain damage, other than dementia, since this is described by Gilhooly in Chapter 7 of this volume. In providing a description of problems which can occur across different types of brain damage, four factors need to be considered — namely pre-onset, onset, the nature of the problems, and changes over time.

Pre-onset factors

It is important to understand the unique set of experiences and circumstances which the family possesses before the onset of any brain damage. Furthermore, it is suggested that to some extent brain damage does not occur at random amongst members of the population.

For example, in genetically transmitted conditions such as Huntington's disease the offspring of an affected parent has a 50 per cent chance of inheritance. In addition, there is a higher than normal incidence of multiple sclerosis amongst close relatives of known sufferers. This means that family members may feel worried about being at risk, as well as having to cope with an affected individual in the family.

Those who suffer a severe head injury may be a special group, in that there is a high preponderance of young males who may have been drinking excessively, have had an above-average number of previous convictions, and may have exhibited other anti-social behaviours. Even if there is not a history of poor premorbid functioning, the person may be young and just developing a career, family and friends at the time of onset, which may cause extra problems of adjustment.

Onset

Some conditions, such as a head injury or a stroke, have a traumatic and rapid onset, whereas others such as Huntington's disease or multiple sclerosis have a gradual onset. As discussed in more detail later, this may have important implications for the way in which the person and the family come to terms with the problems.

Nature of problems

The types of problems that can occur after brain damage are varied, and there are many possible combinations of symptoms. This is true for a given condition such as a stroke, as well as when comparing the effects of different types of brain damage.

With conditions involving a traumatic onset there may be a number of problems which are present at first. Over time there may be recovery of some problems (e.g. language impairment) leaving or even revealing other difficulties (e.g. altered mood). Obviously the reverse may be true of a progressive disorder in that additional deficits may occur over time.

Changes over time

It is important to consider the time after onset of brain damage regardless of whether the condition is progressive or may involve recovery; not only because the direct consequences may vary over time, but also because the family may have particular concerns based upon the time course of the condition. For example, the spouse of someone with a severe head injury may be particularly distressed 1 year after the accident if there is a realisation of the severity and possible persistent nature of the deficits (Rosenbaum and Najenson, 1976).

The duration of the brain damage may also be particularly pertinent for those with a life-threatening or progressive disorder because of the reduction in life expectancy and probable gradual reduction in the quality of life.

Bearing in mind the considerations mentioned above, an outline of the stages involved in adjusting to brain damage will be provided.

GENERAL ISSUES FOLLOWING BRAIN DAMAGE IN THE FAMILY

Initial reaction

The initial shock of learning that someone has had a serious accident, or a stroke, can be devastating for a family. There may be uncertainty about whether the person will live, and about how seriously affected the person may be. Thus the family of someone who has just suffered a severe head injury may sit beside the person for hours without getting any response, whilst anxiously awaiting any sign of movement, and being surrounded by unfamiliar and confusing terminology and technology. Experience of working with families coming to terms with different types of brain damage has emphasised the need that families have for talking with others in a similar situation right from the earliest stages after the onset of the brain damage. For example, the same problem may have been experienced by other families, who can then say how they coped, or they may be able to reassure a family with a recently injured member that a particular problem was a phase which could occur during the person's recovery, but which does not last. Thus the establishment of a contact service with other carers via self-help groups or on an individual basis can be of help (see section on Support Groups for further details). This need may be greatest at the early stage after brain damage, but may diminish and cease if a good recovery is made.

Overcoming uncertainty

Whether the condition involves improvement or deterioration over time, there is likely to be uncertainty about the rate of change, and the type of problems to expect at particular times. One way the professional can help at this time is to give some understanding of what the problems are at a particular point in time, and to monitor progress with particular abilities in order to give guidelines about future recovery or deterioration. With some conditions, such as multiple sclerosis or Huntington's disease, the onset may be very insidious, and the professionals then have the responsibility of reducing uncertainty and providing an accurate diagnosis. Concern about the various symptoms may continue beyond the stage of diagnosis, since with multiple sclerosis the symptoms may remain vague and changeable, with the constant worry of a more general relapse. Furthermore, members of the family of someone with a genetically transmitted disorder such as Huntington's disease may be at risk of having the disease themselves, and therefore may anxiously watch for symptoms in themselves and other family members.

Understanding

A common adage I often hear from relatives, and those with brain damage, is that, 'You don't know what it is like until you have been through it yourself.' This is undoubtedly true, and emphasises how alone families may feel with their problems. They may feel that professionals did not know the person before the brain injury, and thus may describe the person in ways which the family do not recognise.

Friends and relatives may visit and only see the best aspects of the person with brain damage. The lack of obvious problems may mean that these friends do not appreciate the worries and strain felt by the immediate family.

It can also be difficult for the immediate family, and the person with brain damage, to understand the nature of the problems. For example, one relative I know cannot accept that his wife can still read, but has so many problems with even basic skills. Another problem which is often misunderstood is that of dyspraxia, where the connection between the intention and the action is affected. The problem may be misconstrued as laziness, stubbornness or of a hysterical nature, particularly as the person may be unable to carry out an act when requested, but may do so straight away when not pressured.

Another important source of misunderstanding is the emotional state of the affected person. Following brain damage the person may change mood more readily, not only from day to day but also within short periods during the day. This may be difficult to accept, particularly if, for example, episodes of crying are construed by the relative as indicative of depression, which makes the relative upset as well. Unfortunately, the rapid lifting of the mood of the person with brain damage may not be matched by that of the relative, who may remain distraught and also rather bemused by these episodes.

In addition, the person may laugh at simple things which do not appeal to others, and this may become irksome for the family, whereas those in less frequent contact with the person may tolerate or even enjoy such behaviour. This may further alienate the relative from others.

Just as the relative may have difficulty understanding the person with brain damage, so the converse is also true. Firstly, in general those with brain damage tend to under-report problems compared with the reports of carers (McKinlay, Brooks, Bond, Martinage and Marshall, 1981). This may mean that the person does not understand the extent of the problems experienced by the carer. Secondly, those with brain damage may have diminished appreciation of the mood of others and be particularly poor at judging negative emotions such as sadness or anger in others (Jackson and Moffat, 1987). This may be a further cause of frustration since the person may seem surprised if told off, leaving the relative still feeling angry, or possibly then feeling guilty at getting annoyed with the person. Again the carer may remain upset for longer than the person with brain damage.

The lack of understanding by the person and others of the strain involved may mean that the relative feels he or she is being taken for granted.

Wish for a cure

The family may be frustrated and angry with doctors for not continuing to take an interest in the family, and for not being able to provide a cure. In the case of a disorder such as multiple sclerosis, the lack of a known aetiology may result in spurious ideas about causality and a belief that unusual treatments may be beneficial. The family may also feel angry towards the patient in the belief that the person could try harder, and should be highly motivated to seek a cure.

With a recovering condition such as a head injury, the family may maintain hope of a good recovery for many months whilst progress is being achieved. However, it has already been mentioned that perhaps 1 year post-injury the relatives of those with a severe head injury may begin to realise the extent and persistent nature of the problems, and this may prove a crucial time when the feelings of hope could give way to those of resignation, and possibly of helplessness and depression. This is not helped if reports by the family of small improvements are mistrusted by professionals on the assumption that it could be wishful thinking.

Expectations

There is sometimes a tendency for others, including professionals, to see the presence of brain damage in the family as a terrible tragedy, and to think that the carer should feel depressed. This undermines the confidence of the family and can build up a lack of trust, with the hospital staff being worried about whether the person is being properly looked after at home. Conversely, the lack of resources in the hospital may mean that families are dissatisfied with the hospital care, and the hospital may expect the family to cope with behaviour problems that they have been unable to deal with. Unfortunately, some families believe that the problems will all disappear when the person gets home.

Dependence

There may be a difference of opinion between professionals and family members regarding the most appropriate way of working with the person with brain damage. Thus, professionals may emphasise the maintenance and enhancement of the person's independence, which may help the person's recovery in the long term, but does require extra time and effort in the short term. However, the family may prefer a more expedient course of action; for example it may be easier to dress the person than to wait for self-initiated attempts.

The need for some help with tasks can also be a cause of embarrassment and loss of dignity. Some individuals will resist checks or assistance with such tasks as bathing, which can cause considerable friction within a family. The rejection of help may be an indication of a poor acceptance of the problems, as may excessive efforts to equal previous skills, or those of the able-bodied. This is particularly highlighted if the person refuses to discuss the disability or if family members deny that there are any problems.

Another issue is that some families may be worried about the ability of the person, and have fears related to this, such as that the slightest bump on the head could cause further brain damage. Furthermore, the person with brain damage may have lost confidence and be reluctant to attempt activities.

Reduction in activities

Families often report that they have had to give up many activities as a result of caring for someone with severe brain damage. This may be partially due to the person's reduced interests and activities in the home. In addition, contact with others may be diminished, possibly because friends visit less often.

There is some evidence that a reduction in activities may be associated with depression in the carer (Moffat, 1978; Rosenbaum and Najenson, 1976). Thus, the maintenance of established relationships and the formation of new friendships may be important for the well-being of relatives.

Adjusting to disability

It is suggested that it is difficult for the person with brain damage, and also for the relative, to come to terms with the effects of brain damage. Thus the family may be aware of major changes in the personality of the person affected, with families sometimes saying that the person is not the same any more. This feeling of loss of the person has been described as a 'living bereavement', or as a process of 'mobile mourning' (Muir and Haffey, 1984), which emphasises the continual nature of such an adjustment. In other words, firstly there is not a normal bereavement in that the person is still present, albeit changed. Secondly, the problems may change over time and therefore as the family come to terms with one problem this may be replaced by others.

An additional process which may occur amongst family members is that of denial, possibly of the presence or the permanence of disability (Romano, 1974). This may be an appropriate coping mechanism in some ways, but exaggerated and prolonged denial can prevent that person, and other members of the family, from accepting the disability and adopting a more appropriate lifestyle. Denial is particularly likely to occur with regard to impairment of mental ability or altered mood, since the effects may not be immediately obvious.

It may be particularly difficult for someone with brain damage to adjust to his/her own problems because of the wide implications of brain damage, and the special difficulties of coming to terms with them whilst suffering from impaired mental processes. For example, the effects of the loss of communication and of the use of a dominant hand following a severe right-sided stroke has been described as a 'catastrophic reaction' at being unable to do things, particularly when speech is affected (Gainotti, 1983):

Mr D. suffered a stroke which left him with a problem expressing himself, although he could understand what was said to him. He was very frustrated by this problem, and anxiously avoided meeting people. He regained some of his confidence and his fluency of speech by the use of melodic intonation therapy (Sparks, Helm and Albert, 1974), which utilised the preserved sense of rhythm to make his speech more song-like. He became less embarrassed when conversing with his wife, but she tended to speak for him, or provide him with simple 'yes-no' choices in order to circumvent the obvious frustration he exhibited. This resulted in very limited conversations between them, and a shift in the responsibilities for the running of the home from him to her.

Those with brain damage may also experience problems of adjustment caused by the reaction of others. Thus there may be stigma or fear of stigma by the sufferer. For example, a person who has epileptic seizures may have to overcome prejudice about marriage since, until relatively recently in some states in the USA, people with epilepsy were not allowed to marry. Thus it may be useful to provide information and counselling for families so that they feel better able to inform others in an appropriate way.

Strain

The burden of caring refers to the objective difficulties that the relative notices about the dependant, whereas strain can be defined as the measure of the distress felt by the carer.

Generally with the severely head-injured there is a close relationship between the objective burden and the level of strain felt by the carer during the early months after the head injury (McKinlay *et al.*, 1981). The closeness of this relationship decreases after this time for a variety of reasons. Firstly, it is the nature and not the number of problems that matter. Thus there is general agreement in the literature that mood and behaviour disturbances are more likely to be a source of strain to relatives than impairment of physical functioning (Bond, 1975). Furthermore, this is true not only during the first year after injury but also in longer-term follow-up studies in which behavioural problems continue to be a significant burden for the relatives (Lezak, 1978; Lezak, Cosgrove, O'Brien and Wooster, 1980; and Thomsen, 1981).

. Secondly, families may vary in the way in which they construe the same problem. Thus one carer may help a person with dressing with enthusiasm, whereas another may find the same task a chore. The accumulation of these small chores or hassles may be a contributor to psychological symptoms (Kanner, Coyne, Schaefer and Lazarus, 1981; Monroe, 1983). For example, activities which might have been uplifting of mood previously, such as going out, may now have become a hassle, and require planning, and hence no longer be uplifting of mood.

As an indication of the level of stress experienced by the families of someone with a head injury, the spouses show relatively high rates of divorce and of illness (Panting and Merry, 1972), with a high level of depression (Rosenbaum and Najenson, 1976). Often the strain is not confined to a spouse: for example the blood relative of someone with Huntington's disease may also be highly stressed by the knowledge of being at risk of the disorder. This at-risk group also show a relatively high rate of divorce, and also of alcohol problems, child neglect, and psychiatric disorder (Oliver, 1970a,b). In one study, about half of those at risk said that they would consider suicide if they developed Huntington's disease (Wexler, 1979).

The burden of caring may mean that the carer feels exhausted by the extra duties, and possibly becomes disorganised. There may be some underlying resentment at being expected to cope, and some wish to be cared for.

Role adjustment

Pre-onset family characteristics

The amount and type of change in role for the brain-damaged person and the family depends upon the nature of the pre-injury relationships. For example, families in which the wife has multiple sclerosis generally report fewer problems than those in which the husband is a sufferer. This appears to be related to the feeling of loss of the male breadwinning role. Another observation made amongst families with a person with multiple sclerosis is that spouses who have been more satisfied with their relationships tend to fight the illness label longer, whereas those who had a less satisfactory relationship accept the illness label more readily, and are more likely to dissociate themselves from their partner both physically and mentally, and eventually get divorced (Simons, 1984).

There is some suggestion that the head-injured living with parents may be tolerated more readily than a head-injured person living with a spouse (Panting and Merry, 1972; Thomsen, 1974). This may be because childish behaviour is more readily tolerated by parents, and also the expectations of the person are different.

Changes in the responsibilities of family members

The person with brain damage may become depressed at having to give up duties, and the response of the carer may vary, such that some carers may enjoy taking on extra responsibilities, with the family perhaps finding that it has 'a new captain but maybe an unwilling crew'. Conversely, the carer may be reluctant to take on the responsibilities, and the person with brain damage may be unable to manage, resulting in the family being analogous to 'a ship without a captain'. For example this may occur if the condition is progressive and the carer is reluctant to take over the management of affairs. It could also occur if the person has access to large quantities of money following compensation, which may be unwisely spent.

The process of initial adjustment mentioned above may require reversal again if the person with brain damage makes a significant recovery. This process of adjustment and re-adjustment may proceed smoothly if the affected person makes a reasonably rapid and complete recovery. However, problems may arise if the adjusted roles have been established for some time, and have become fossilised.

Thus the carer may have found it easier to help the person to get dressed rather than to encourage independence. There may also be an understandable mistrust of the person's ability to manage again.

Permanency of role changes

It may be particularly difficult for young couples to accept the possible permanent effects of brain damage. Thus, in the case of the slow and partial recovery after a severe head injury, the wife may not be clear about the long-term prospects for many months after the accident when the more permanent deficits are known.

For those who care for someone with a more progressive or permanent condition the process of adjustment may be rather insidious, and gradually become totally time-consuming. This may be accepted with good grace at the time, but for some carers the ending of such a commitment may be traumatic. This could occur following the death or hospitalisation of the dependent person. The long-term effects of caring can be seen amongst some members of the National Association of Carers and their Elderly Dependants, who as single women have had little opportunity to maintain or develop relationships and interests outside of this caring role. As one recently bereaved carer told me, 'It is like being let out of prison, and the only feeling is a wish to be let back inside again.'

For those carers who do not expect to outlive their dependent relatives, such as parents of a young head-injured person, there may be concern about what will happen to the person in the long term. This often reflects a natural preference for family and home-based existence, rather than any form of hospital care.

Broader family roles

The effects of brain damage may have significant ripples throughout the family. For example, in a number of families I am working with, tolerance of the children's behaviour by the parent with a head injury is limited. The affected parent then vacillates between excessive disciplining of the children and withdrawal and regret. The unaffected parent then has to mediate between the two parties, sometimes construing the behaviour of all concerned as childlike. There is some evidence with regard to the effects upon siblings in that the school performance of the sibling of a head-injured person is affected for the year post-injury (Cunning, 1976). An additional effect upon the family is that the relationship with in-laws may become more strained (Rosenbaum and Najenson, 1976).

With regard to multiple sclerosis, it is suggested that the parents are poor at judging the effects upon the children of having someone in the family with this disorder. Child behaviour problems do occur in about one-fifth of families, and there may be concern about the level of physical care for the children (Braham, Houser, Cline and Posner, 1975). However, generally the children are well adjusted, and may show greater anxiety about the family than about themselves.

The acquisition of brain damage by one member of the family not only requires adjustment in terms of pre-onset relationships, but also has important implications for the future plans of the family. For example, it has been found that about one-quarter of those at risk of Huntington's disease go on to have children after they have learned about the hereditary nature of the disease. The choice of having a child may be a positive one in that there is a chance the child does not inherit the condition. Furthermore, even if he or she does inherit the disorder there may be 30 or more years of normal life to be enjoyed. For example, Woody Guthrie (the American folk singer who inspired others such as Bob Dylan) died of Huntington's disease, and his wife has aptly asked whether or not this talented man should have been born.

The impact on the family of most forms of brain damage is usually to diminish future objectives. This may include a reduction in socioeconomic status through the loss of the breadwinning role by the injured person and also the carer in severe cases. For young people there is the loss of opportunities, such as not resuming education, and perhaps having diminished prospects for marriage. Older families may also experience losses, such as being unable to enjoy intended retirement plans. These types of loss may leave all concerned with a feeling of being cheated. It is important for professionals who are working with these families to be aware of the original wishes and hopes of the family, so that the full impact of new plans can be understood.

Thus it is the challenge of work with the brain-damaged to help the person and his/her family cope at home, and also to make suitable alternative provision for the brain-damaged person in the event that the family are no longer able to cope on a short- or long-term basis.

The next section will describe some of the more common problems after brain damage, and how families can cope with these difficulties.

GENERAL STRATEGIES FOR COPING

The definition of coping given by Lazarus and Folkman (1984) is that coping involves 'constantly changing cognitive and behavioural efforts to manage specific external and/or internal demands that are appraised as taxing or exceeding the resources of the person'. This definition emphasises the need to consider the diverse and changeable ways in which people may attempt to cope with their own interpretations of different situations.

Various taxonomies of coping have been suggested, with a general distinction being made between problem-focused and emotion-focused responses (Folkman and Lazarus, 1980). However, in most instances both types of coping are used simultaneously when coping with a particular stressful encounter. Furthermore, it is not possible to state the proportion of problem- to emotion-focused strategies that is appropriate for a particular type of stressful episode.

Although there is a considerable literature on coping, there is little on the ways in which families cope with acquired brain damage other than dementia. Therefore the following description of situational factors and strategies used by families is drawn mainly from clinical experience.

Situational factors

The general style of relationship between family members may have a bearing upon the ways in which families cope. As a general dimension one can consider that families vary in terms of how emotionally close or distant the members are. Taking the extremes, and beginning with a very close couple, one of whom is brain-damaged, the typical pattern of relationship may consist of an over-functioning relative and an under-functioning dependent person. The couple may withdraw from others and may be reluctant to seek professional services or share responsibilities with professionals, and may tend to retain rather fixed ideas and routines. The task for this type of family may be to recognise the stress upon the carer, and to share responsibilities.

Amongst families who may be typified as having a distant type of relationship between members, there may be a somewhat different style of coping. Typically such families may have had less intense emotional relationships and family members may be physically further away from one another. Family members may be reluctant to take on responsibilities themselves, and be keen to achieve short-term solutions rather than to work towards longer-term alternatives.

It is important to consider the full family when looking at styles of coping, since issues such as the sharing of power may have impli-cations for all concerned. For example, an older couple may have to relinquish some responsibilities if one partner is incapacitated, and the children of that couple may then be expected to take on extra responsibility. Another reason for looking at the whole family is to check the way in which the family copes. There may be apparent order in one set of relationships, but this may be achieved by distortions in other relationships, such as scapegoating certain members, whether this is the brain-damaged person, the carer or another family member. For example, an offspring of a person with brain damage may be seen to act out the stress experienced by the family, and is scapegoated as the deviant member of the family.

A general principle that is important in work with the brain-damaged is the facilitation of ways of coping. It appears that sugges-tions are not followed through, not because of resistance to coopera-tion but because the demands of looking after someone with brain damage use up the resources of the carer, which makes it difficult to carry out intentions.

The following is an attempt to define and categorise the rich and varied ways of coping I have observed, or which have been described to me by families.

Classification of styles of coping

Practical and motivational problem-solving

The general style which describes this type of coping is to 'have a go', in that there is an effort to try to make things work. A variety of more specific strategies can be subsumed under this heading:

Rise to the challenge.
Maintain enthusiasm.
Maintain expectations of the person.
Make a plan and follow it.
Break the task down into small achievable parts.
Look for small improvements, and generally alter aspirations.
Foresee problems and seek ways of coping or avoiding them.
Seek innovative ways of coping.
Seek alternative sources of gratification.

During the early years after brain damage, there may be a tendency for families and affected individuals to respond with anger and increased motivation to overcome any resistance to freedom of action (Wortman and Brehm, 1975). This type of 'reactance' is often strong amongst those who have recovered, or are trying to recover, to a greater extent than was originally predicted. The determination may be maintained for many months or years, but the realisation of a somewhat uncontrollable outcome, and the effort involved in making small progress, may lead to a gradual reduction in motivation, with increased passivity and depression. Counselling individuals and families at this stage may help them to adjust and seek altered aspirations and alternative means of gratification.

Diplomatic problem-solving

In order to manage effectively the carer of someone with brain damage may need to be a good diplomat. This is because the person with brain damage may readily take offence or become stubborn if something is not presented in an acceptable way. The following strategies can be considered under this heading:

Not act hastily.
Appeal to the person's good nature.
Be sensitive to the person's mood that day.
Reduce the person's anxiety, perhaps by not telling him or her until the last minute about plans which it is known would cause worry.

Reappraisal

This can be described as a cognitive and emotional strategy, in which there is a readjustment of values:

Rethink what is important in life.
Become more emotionally detached, often noticeable by the use of terms such as 'they' by relatives when referring to their brain-damaged family members.
Not think too much about the situation.
Look on the bright side of things.
Not get upset about little things.
Take things one day at a time.
Recognise that episodes of mood or behaviour disturbance pass quickly.
Recognise that problems may not be addressed at the carer personally.
Recognise that the person may not be, or at least may not remain, as upset or distressed as the carer following upsets.

Collective coping

The value of peer contact is that it enables people in similar circumstances to share and compare experiences:

Gain a sense of collective coping, in that the problem is shared with others.

Comparison with others may help a carer to feel that there is always someone worse off.

Associate with powerful others. For example, a relative may be able to gain the goodwill of a brain-damaged family member by saying that a particular activity needs to be carried out at the request of a respected other.

Seek social support.

Loyalty

There is a sense of commitment to the person, and a desire to maintain the dignity of the individual as he or she was before the brain damage. Despite the lack of appreciation by the dependent person of the efforts of the carer, the latter may preserve this sense of loyalty by:

A commitment to caring. The carer may reason that the dependent relative would have done the same if the situation had been reversed. Furthermore, the carer may state that, as they have had a good life together, the brain-damaged person deserves the care and the carer owes this commitment to him or her.

Maintaining respect for the person.

Avoiding making the person a 'patient', for example by maintaining the person's independence.

Thinking back to good times prior to the onset of brain damage.

Catharsis

It may be very important for family members to be able to express their emotions by:

Crying.

Laughter and retaining a sense of humour.

Losing temper.

Discharging energy effectively.

Expressing self creatively.

The general coping strategies mentioned above may be used when dealing with some of the more specific problems following brain damage. However, as outlined below, a more specific set of coping strategies can be identified for dealing with specific deficits, such as memory problems.

WAYS OF COPING WITH SPECIFIC PROBLEMS FOLLOWING BRAIN DAMAGE

Memory problems

The range of everyday memory problems which may occur following brain damage depends upon the nature and severity of the brain damage. Some of the more common examples include problems with concentration, forgetting day-to-day events, repeating questions or statements, and becoming muddled about the time (year, month or day), as well as about the passage of time. The following are a set of tips to help cope with memory problems:

Memory aids

Signposts, clocks, reminder boards, diaries, calendars and newspapers may help to compensate for difficulty with remembering.

Reality orientation

Repeatedly supplying information which the person has forgotten may help to make sense of what is going on (Holden and Woods, 1982). This should be stated in as short and natural a way as possible.

Tips about communication

Eye contact and possibly touch may help to attract and maintain attention, as may sitting close to the person. Speech should be slow and clear, using short simple sentences which should be repeated if necessary. The person should be encouraged to repeat what has been said, and to respond appropriately. Conversations should be kept specific and objects or photographs may help in this respect, as may stimulation of all of the senses. Confused thinking may be helped by following any of the following suggestions:

1. If possible, tactfully disagree but do not argue with the person.
2. Change the subject and try to discuss something specific.

3. Agree to take a break and to resume the conversation later.
4. Acknowledge how the person may be feeling from what has been said, whilst ignoring the direct content.

Reduce distractions

Avoid talking if there are other things going on at the same time (e.g. the radio or television are on).

Make life simpler

This can be done by maintaining a daily and weekly routine, and by keeping things in the same place.

Limit the choice when dressing

For example, it can be helpful to lay clothes out in order, and if necessary to put all the other clothes out of the way, perhaps even locking the wardrobe.

Limit the choice when eating

If the person gets muddled during mealtimes it may be necessary to take away any condiments following the main course. Leaving the dirty dishes around for a while after a meal has been eaten may help to demonstrate to the person that a meal has just been consumed.

Losing and hiding things

It may be possible to reduce the number of potential hiding places by keeping valuables out of sight, and locking any unused drawers or cupboards. Keep a spare set of household keys in case the original ones get lost.

Wandering

If the person appears agitated and restless then a less stimulating environment, or the opportunity to withdraw to a quieter area, may be helpful. Alternatively, if the person will only engage in an activity for a few minutes then he or she may be able to take part in what is going on (e.g. dusting).

Locking the doors, and the use of an identity bracelet or name tag sewn into the clothes, may help others to assist if the person does become lost.

Avoid stress for the memory-impaired person

Even simple tasks may require additional effort after brain damage, and tiredness, worry or low mood may all affect performance.

With some conditions the memory problem may improve over time, and hence the problem may resolve itself. If the memory problem is progressive, then the distress that accompanies insight may lessen as the person becomes less aware of instances of memory failure.

Recognising the strain upon others

The reduced quality of conversations resulting from poor memory may be upsetting, and constant repetitions or questions may test the patience of the most saintly individual. It is generally not worth arguing a point with someone who has a serious memory problem.

One consolation is that if the carer does get upset with the person, then he/she may have forgotten the incident very shortly afterwards, and it is only the carer who is left feeling upset and possibly unnecessarily guilty.

Language impairment

Impairment of some aspects of language may occur following brain damage, typically if there is right-sided hemiplegia and damage to the left side of the brain.

Successful adaptation to the impaired language of one member of a family seems to rely upon encouraging the person to maintain activities and independence, rather than treating the person in a patronising way. For the family members it is a matter of allowing time for the person to respond, not being critical of the responses the person makes, the sharing of humour, and recognising that raising the voice does not help. The seeking out of adult rather than child-like materials can also be helpful. Since many dysphasics may also have some impairment of memory, allowance may also be needed for this.

It is hard for relatives to see a person struggle to find the right words, and hence they may understandably help the person out, or perhaps only ask simple questions. Training relatives in an experimental situation in how to maximise the speech of their spouse has not always generalised to the home (Diller, Ben-Yishay, Weinberg, Goodkin and Gordon, 1974). There was some indication from this research that the quality of the husband-and-wife relationship before the stroke had a bearing upon whether families could continue with the encouragement they initially carried out in the experimental situation.

Hemi-inattention

A problem that sometimes occurs after brain damage is the ignoring of one side of the body and of what is happening on that side. Thus, right-sided brain damage may result in ignoring the left-hand side. Neglect is particularly common during the early stages after a stroke, and often improves rapidly during the first month. The person may bump into things on the left, eat from only one side of the plate, have difficulty reading, and appear to deny or ignore an affected limb (Keenan, Kapur and Moffat, 1986).

Families may be able to help by encouraging the person to be aware of the problem, since denial is often strong. A simple strategy is to encourage the person to turn the head to the left. In addition, sitting on the person's left and encouraging attention to the left may be of value. Activities need to take account of the neglect, and therefore simple visual material may be better at first, such as large-print books, and the finger used to trace across the page whilst reading. A border on the left of the page may be a helpful reminder.

Frontal lobe impairments

Damage to the frontal lobes may impair a variety of complex skills, since the person may not be able to learn from experience or see the consequences of actions. In addition, there may be a lack of initiative, and sometimes a behaviour may be repeated over and over (perseveration). These problems are a major challenge in rehabilitation, particularly as they may be accompanied by mood changes, sometimes of disinhibition, or alternatively of severe anxiety.

Providing a clear structure for the person may help, such as a list of instructions to follow. This can give general principles such as 'check what you have to do next', as well as specific instructions. Sometimes perseveration may be circumvented by interrupting or startling the person. Coping with the mood changes associated with brain damage, including frontal impairment, are discussed in the next section.

Mood and behaviour disturbance

Changes in the personality and conduct of the person after brain damage appear to be amongst the hardest for patients and especially

257

relatives to come to terms with. Thus, Brooks and Aughton (1979) found that the best predictors of the subjective burden for relatives 6 months after head injury were the brain-injured person's childish behaviour, loss of interest, changes in sex life, depression, and tension/anxiety.

Relatives seem to feel particularly aggrieved at the loss of the reciprocal relationship, when the person with brain injury appears indifferent, with less feelings or empathy towards the partner. This contributes to the feeling of loss of a confidant, and difficulty of open emotional exchange with the partner.

Coping with mood and behaviour problems seems to rely upon a variety of strategies, particularly those involving reappraisal and diplomatic problem-solving, as described earlier.

The way the carer perceives the altered mood is important: it could be seen in at least four possible ways. First, there may be some degree of denial, with the relative saying, for example, that the person was always rather irritable. This may have been partially true, but there may be an attempt to minimise pathological mood disturbance. It may be important to separate out the effects of brain damage from earlier behaviour, since this can provide a clearer understanding of the objectives of rehabilitation, and reduce the risk of attempting to remodel the person beyond what is reasonable.

A second perception might be that mood disturbance is natural under the circumstances, an expression of the frustration at not being able to function as before. This form of empathy may be appropriate, but an over-forgiving attitude may develop in which excessive behaviour is tolerated.

A third approach may be to attribute the behaviour to the brain damage. This may help because unpleasant behaviour directed at the relative may then not be taken personally, and a forgiving attitude may be taken. Perceiving this as out of character may also mean that positive action may be taken to bring the behaviour under control, such as taking a firm attitude to such behaviour, or using professional advice, or treatment such as medication. In addition, strategies for ignoring the behaviour may be brought into play. Furthermore, there may be a willingness to perceive apparent mood expression by the dependent person as not necessarily representative of the mood felt by the dependent person. For example crying may not mean that the person is particularly low in mood.

A final perception is that difficult behaviour is deliberate and under voluntary control. This may enable a family to set limits for acceptable behaviour.

In order to cope effectively a family may need to consider each of these four perspectives and not perceive all behaviour in terms of only some of them.

ASSISTING COPING AMONGST FAMILIES

This chapter has considered a number of problems which may be associated with brain damage, and outlined various ways in which families might cope. It has been suggested that the family has to adjust to the primary effects of brain damage, such as memory problems, and also to the possibly wide and prolonged consequences of having someone in the family suffering from brain damage.

It is important to state that having someone in the family with brain damage does not necessarily cause disruption to the family, and therefore the problems mentioned earlier are not inevitable nor likely to occur in all families. Occasionally improvements can be reported following a severe head injury. Increased assertiveness is an example. This might be directly attributable to the effects of the head injury, or to the further development of the person during the long process of recovery. Thus, Oddy and Humphrey (1980) found little sign of family disruption two years after one member had suffered a severe head injury. The optimistic findings of this study probably result from the relatively mildly injured sample, with disruption being least in those with a duration of post-traumatic amnesia, or confusion follow-ing the accident, of less than a week. Similarly, Bishop, Epstein, Keitner, Miller and Srinivasan (1986) found no differences on a variety of measures between control families and those with a member who had suffered a stroke one year beforehand. On the other hand, Williams and Freer (1986) did find disruptions within families with a dysphasic member, and noted that the spouses of the more mildly impaired were significantly less well informed. This suggests that dif-ferent types of counselling may be needed to suit the nature and severity of problems in the family following brain damage of one member.

Four main ways of helping can be identified, starting with sup-port groups for families with similar problems.

Support groups

Most of the self-help groups for families with a brain-injured member do provide local forums for families to meet. The popularity and rapid

259

growth of these self-help organisations emphasise the importance that families place upon membership and meeting other people. Certainly, the value of meeting others may be in terms of collective coping described earlier, in which carers feel that they are not alone with a problem. Furthermore, there may be a degree of social comparison involved in gauging how each carer feels he or she is coping. This may give a sense of relative competence by comparison with others. However, there are virtually no properly controlled trials of the value of support groups. Furthermore, the unselective and unstructured nature of many such groups means that carers may not model themselves upon experienced and effective carers; and group members may not identify their own deficits in coping, nor attempt to improve their range and depth of coping skills. In some cases membership of a special group may begin to replace contacts with other members of the community.

If structured groups are being considered it may be important to provide a suitable mix of group members, who share similar experiences. For example, younger carers often feel they have been cheated of their present and future plans, and that older carers and dependants have already had a more complete and good life together. Therefore, group members should include an appropriate mix of younger and older members, or alternatively groups should be specific to either young or older carers. Groups can also be divided into those carers who are coping with the early stages after onset, and those who have been coping for a long time. This may help to lessen the somewhat unsympathetic attitude I have observed in groups in which those who have been coping for longer may be intolerant of problems expressed by the less experienced. This unsympathetic attitude is also a function of how often these issues have been discussed in the group in the past, with tolerance being less if the same concerns have been discussed at length recently. Although a degree of homogeneity of group members and their experiences is important, excessive homogeneity may have the adverse effect of not providing sufficient variety of experience to enable group members to state how they have coped with particular problems.

Information

In the case of many types of brain damage, particularly head injury (Rosenthal *et al.*, 1983), there appears to be a strongly felt need for improved communication with doctors, and for more information.

This can be done as part of the normal routine of the team working with the family, but the relatives of the head-injured generally feel that this is inadequate. The self-help organisations do provide a generalised service via the range of information they produce. Furthermore, some self-help groups mix their programme between informal social functions, and structured meetings with a speaker and discussion on particular topics. Some hospitals are beginning to provide formal sessions for relatives, although this is better suited to the larger or more specialised services in order to provide regular and timely advice.

Having someone in the family with severe brain damage may give the family a new mission in life, such that they become recognised as the real experts at coping, not the specialist professionals. For example, the family may notice that some progress is occurring before the professional does, which once confirmed may enable the family to feel that 'I told you so'. Particularly at the later stages after brain damage, the family may have to act as their own advocates for services and benefits, since it is rare to find professionals who maintain a long-standing commitment to the family. This is unfortunate in that many families already feel over-burdened and isolated. It is recommended that professionals, particularly general practitioners, should adopt a reaching-out policy in order to ensure that families are seen regularly and services and entitlements are offered to them.

Professionals can also foster a more independent spirit amongst families by being available when required, and by listening and responding to their needs, whilst keeping the responsibility for decision-making with the family.

Training in coping

Reliance upon the model of education mentioned above assumes that difficulty with coping is partly a function of lack of information. This may be so, but in some cases information may not be enough, and relatives may benefit from more formal training in coping. Training carers in specific skills may consist of ways of coping for themselves, e.g. learning relaxation to cope with stress (Levine, Gendron, Dastour, Poitras, Sirota, Barzaa and Davis, 1983); or may be in terms of ways of influencing the behaviour of the brain-damaged person. In our own work the former aim has been pursued via structured support groups (Trigg, 1984); and the latter aim by training carers to carry out rehabilitation programmes with the dependent person at home

(Moffat, in press). It appears that the success of a home-based therapy relies upon the combination of a remediable problem, a person with good insight and motivation, and a keen carer, with a good relationship between the family members.

Attitudes

The final approach, which is related to the points mentioned above, relies upon the attitude of the family. Certainly, directly experiencing or living with someone who has brain damage is likely to involve major readjustments, and at times may require considerable tolerance and patience. The carer may lose some feelings towards the person, which may be replaced by other feelings such as empathy and possibly sympathy for the person.

Unwittingly, the person with brain damage may show only limited appreciation of the efforts of others, which means that family members have to rely more upon their own source of encouragement. This unmet need of being appreciated and cared for should be acknowledged and provided for. For example, we arrange monthly outings for carers who otherwise have little opportunity to get out and enjoy themselves.

With regard to those who have acquired brain damage it is important to look at their assets as well as their deficits in skills, and to maintain an interest in the person.

Finally, families may be able to look back over past events and reinterpret them in the light of new information. For example, initially the onset of brain damage may be construed as due to hard work; whereas later knowledge may change this attribution to something outside of the person's own making, which might ease any potential guilt the carer experienced.

What may be important within a family is not simply the individual style of coping, but also the shared nature of aims. Thus the shared notion that the prognosis is good, or bad, may be more efficacious than where such views are discordant. The recognition that support from others is available, and the willingness to use this, may be positively related to coping. Important within this may be the ability to express feelings, and have these feelings endorsed by others. This goes back to an earlier point that families sometimes feel that 'You don't know what it is like unless you have experienced it yourself.' It is the recognition of this that makes the need for empathic understanding of the ways in which families cope with brain damage all the more challenging and worthwhile.

Acknowledgement

I should like to thank the Head Injuries Rehabilitation Trust for their financial support between 1980 and 1982, which provided the opportunity to work closely with individuals who had suffered a head injury, and their families.

REFERENCES

Bishop, D.S., Epstein, N.B., Keitner, G.I., Miller, I.,W. and Srinivasan, S.V. (1986) Stroke, morale, family functioning, health status, and functional capacity, *Archives of Physical Medicine and Rehabilitation, 67*, 84–7

Bond, M.R. (1975) Assessment of the psychosocial outcome after severe head injury. In *Outcome of severe damage to the central nervous system*, CIBA Foundation Symposium 34, Elsevier, Amsterdam, pp. 141–58

Braham, S., Houser, H.B., Cline, A. and Posner, M. (1975) Evaluation of the social needs of non-hospitalised chronically ill persons: a study of 47 patients with multiple sclerosis, *Journal of Chronic Diseases, 28*, 401–19

Brooks, D.N. and Aughton, M.E. (1979) Psychological consequences of blunt head injury, *International Rehabilitation Medicine, 1*, 160–5

Cunning, J.E. (1976) Emotional aspects of head trauma in children, *Rehabilitation Literature, 37*, 335

Diller, L., Ben-Yishay, Y., Weinberg, J., Goodkin, R. and Gordon, W. (1974) *Studies in cognition and rehabilitation in hemiplegia*, New York University Medical Center Rehabilitation Monograph 50, NYU Medical Center, New York

Folkman, S. and Lazarus, R.S. (1980) An analysis of coping in a middle-aged community sample, *Journal of Health and Social Behaviour, 21*, 219–39

Gainotti, G. (1983) Laterality of affect: the emotional behavior of right and left brain damaged patients. In M.S. Myslobodsky (ed.), *Hemisyndromes: psychobiology, neurology, psychiatry*, Academic Press, New York.

Holden, U.P. and Woods, R.T. (1982) *Reality orientation; psychological approaches to the confused elderly*, Churchill Livingstone, London

Jackson, M.F. and Moffat, N.J. (1987) Impaired emotional recognition following severe head injury, *Cortex* (in press)

Kanner, A.D., Coyne, J.C., Schaefer, C. and Lazarus, R.S. (1981) Comparison of two modes of stress measurement: daily hassles and uplifts versus major life events, *Journal of Behavioral Medicine, 4*, 1–39

Keenan, E., Kapur, N. and Moffat, N.J. (forthcoming) The relationship between unilateral visual neglect and everyday neglect behaviours in patients with right brain damage (Submitted for publication)

Lazarus, R. and Folkman, S. (1984) *Stress, appraisal and coping*, Springer,

New York

Levine, N.B. , Gendron, C.E., Dastour, D.P., Poitras, L.R., Sirota, S.E., Barzaa, S.L. and Davis, J.C. (1983) Supporter endurance training: a manual for trainers, *Clinical Gerontologist, 2*, 15–23

Lezak, M.D. (1978) Living with the characterologically altered brain injured patient, *Journal of Clinical Psychiatry, 39*, 592–8

Lezak, M., Cosgrove, J.N., O'Brien, K. and Wooster, K. (1980) Relationship between personality disorders, social disturbances and physical disability following traumatic brain injury. Paper presented at Eighth Annual Meeting of International Neuropsychological Society, San Francisco. February

McKinlay, W.W., Brooks, D.N., Bond, M.R., Martinage, D.P. and Marshall, M.M. (1981) The short term outcome of severe blunt head injury as reported by the relatives of the head injured person, *Journal of Neurology, Neurosurgery and Psychiatry, 44*, 527–33

Moffat, N.J. (1978) Reported changes in mood, behaviour and family life associated with a severe head injury. Unpublished dissertation, University of Exeter

Moffat, N.J. (in press) Home based cognitive rehabilitation with the elderly. In L.W. Poon, D.C. Rubin and B.A. Wilson (eds), *Everyday cognition in adult and late life*, Cambridge University Press, Cambridge

Monroe, S.C. (1983) Major and minor life events as predictors of psychological distress: further issues and findings, *Journal of Behavioral Medicine, 6*, 189–205

Muir, G.A. and Haffey, W.J. (1984) Psychological and neuropsychological interventions in the mobile mourning process. In B.A. Edelstein and E.T. Couture (eds), *Behavioral assessment and rehabilitation of the traumatically brain-damaged*, Plenum, New York

Oddy, M. and Humphrey, M. (1980) Social recovery during the year following severe head injury, *Journal of Neurology, Neurosurgery and Psychiatry, 43*, 798–802

Oliver, J.E. (1970a) Huntington's chorea in Northamptonshire, *British Journal of Psychiatry, 116*, 241–53

Oliver, J.E. (1970b) Socio-psychiatric consequences of Huntington's disease, *British Journal of Psychiatry, 116*, 255–8

Panting, A. and Merry, P. (1972) The long term rehabilitation of severe head injuries with particular reference to the need for social and medical support for the patient's family, *Rehabilitation, 38*, 33–7

Romano, M.D. (1974) Family response to traumatic head injury, *Scandinavian Journal of Rehabilitation Medicine, 6*, 1–4

Rosenbaum, M. and Najenson, T. (1976) Changes in life patterns and symptoms of low mood as reported by wives of severely brain-injured soldiers, *Journal of Consulting and Clinical Psychology, 44*, 881–8

Rosenthal, M., Griffiths, E.R., Bond, M.R. and Miller, J.D. (eds.) (1983) *Rehabilitation of the head-injured adult*, F.A. Davis, Philadelphia

Simons, A.F. (1984) Problems of providing support for people with multiple sclerosis and their families. In A.F. Simons (ed.), *Multiple sclerosis: psychological and social aspects,* Heinemann Medical Books, London

Sparks, R.W., Helm, N. and Albert, M. (1974) Aphasia rehabilitation resulting from melodic intonation therapy, *Cortex, 10*, 303–16

Thomsen, I.V. (1974) The patient with severe head injury and his family, *Scandinavian Journal of Rehabilitation Medicine, 6*, 180–3

Thomsen, I.V. (1981) Neuropsychological treatment and longterm follow-up in an aphasic patient with very severe head trauma, *Journal of Clinical Neuropsychology, 3*, 43–51

Trigg, A. (1984) An evaluation of a relative support group. Dissertation for British Psychology Society Diploma in Clinical Psychology

Wexler, N.S. (1979) Genetic Russian roulette: the experience of being at risk for Huntington's disease. In S. Kessler (ed.), *Genetic counseling: psychological dimensions*, Academic Press, New York

Williams, S.E. and Freer, C.A. (1986) Aphasia: its effects on marital relationships, *Archives of Physical Medicine and Rehabilitation, 67*, 250–2

Wortman, C.B. and Brehm, J.W. (1975) Responses to uncontrollable outcomes: an integration of reactance theory and the learned helplessness model. In L. Berkowitz (ed.) *Advances in experimental social psychology*, Vol. 8, Academic Press, New York

12

Integration: A General Account of Families Coping with Disorder

Jim Orford

It has been an exhilarating experience, as editor of this volume, to receive the contributory chapters one by one and to see the commonalities emerge. Although there are intriguing differences of emphasis in the ways in which different authors have approached their tasks, the areas of overlap are large, as I had hoped. The subjects which constitute the separate chapters of this book have generally been treated separately in the past. This is, I believe, short-sighted, since each area of expertise has much to offer the others. Collectively, rather than separately, our level of knowledge and understanding is higher, and our ability to devise effective interventions is greater.

This chapter aims to contribute to a collective understanding of families coping with psychological disorder or chronic physical illness, by attempting to integrate the findings and suggestions of the foregoing chapters. It is divided into two parts. The first part offers a description of the common experience of coping with disorder or illness in the family, a description that should be recognisable by those concerned with any one of a range of disorders or handicaps, whether it be renal failure, haemophilia, depression, or excessive drinking, and whether the person affected is a child, a partner, a parent, or a grandparent.

The second part of the chapter will focus on the 'helpers' — a word used broadly here to include all those who are in a special position to help families by virtue of their special expertise or their position in a helping agency. This broad group includes voluntary as well as statutory organisations and many people without formal training in one of the recognised health or social service professions. This second part of the chapter will bring together the many criticisms that have been made of the professionals' negative attitudes and lack of response to families. It will also summarise the suggestions that chapter authors have made about constructive ways in which families can be assisted towards more effective coping.

I. THE NATURE OF THE EXPERIENCE FOR FAMILY MEMBERS

If one feature of the earlier chapters of this book were to be picked out for particular commendation it would surely be the insightful descriptions which they provide of the nature of the experience of living in a family where one member has schizophrenia, Alzheimer's disease, or anorexia nervosa, where one member is violent, or where a family member has any one of the other problems considered in this book. The following is an attempt to bring together those elements that appear to be common to these experiences. This will be done under three headings: the personal, the family, and the extended family and wider community.

The personal experience

Words such as 'stress' and 'burden' are used repeatedly in this book. Indeed several authors remark that the burden of caring or coping has been falling even more heavily upon families in recent years as a result of treatments which prolong life or which control more severe symptoms, and because of a policy — enlightened but backed up with scarce resources — of community care. This point is made by Pahl and Quine, who find that mentally handicapped children at home are comparable to those living in hospital in terms of level of disabilities, and have rather more disability than those living in residential homes; by Nichols, who refers to the way in which families are required to cope with long-term illness, disability or disfigurement once the hospital has successfully carried out short-term treatment and the case is effectively 'closed'; and by Birchwood and Smith, writing of the family burden of coping with schizophrenia.

Practical hardships

Much of the burden which is described is of a very practical kind: it constitutes the 'objective' burden (Kuipers), which is so easily overlooked by health professionals. Financial hardship is a source of stress to which several authors refer. Constant worry about money may be the result of the principal wage-earner's loss of earnings due to depression (Kuipers) or schizophrenia (Birchwood and Smith),

267

because money is being used to finance excessive drinking (McCrady and Hay), or because care for a chronically ill or handicapped family member involves the family in greater expense or because the principal carer (usually a wife or mother) is more restricted in her ability to obtain outside employment, or because a family wage earner feels less able to take on overtime or shift work (Pahl and Quine). Dobash and Dobash also describe the way in which money matters constitute one of the long-standing family disagreements leading to wife abuse.

Accommodation may become more of a problem than it would otherwise have been for a family responsible for specialised treatments at home, such as renal dialysis, which require bulky apparatus or peace and quiet (Nichols), for parents with a mentally handicapped and perhaps disruptive child (Pahl and Quine), or for an abused wife seeking an escape from a violent husband (Dobash and Dobash). Financial and accommodation difficulties constitute an important part of the scale of adversity which Pahl and Quine find to be related to level of stress in the carer.

There may be other, very practical, ways in which a disorder, illness, or disability places an extra stress on the family. One of these, mentioned by a number of authors, is disturbance of sleep. Another is interference with a family's normal dietary habits. Family members' sleep may be disrupted because of the nature of a disorder or illness (e.g. a depressed person waking in the night, or the night wanderings of an elderly confused person), because of pain or distress associated with illness or with treatment (Eiser), or, with some handicapped children (Pahl and Quine), as an extension of the pattern of night-time disruption expected when caring for infants. Whatever its origins sleep disturbance is probably of major importance in creating feelings of exhaustion, lack of energy, and hopelessness in family members. Gilhooly refers to its effects as 'devastating', and Pahl and Quine found the highest stress scores in mothers whose children were wakeful at night.

Eiser makes particular mention of adjustments that may be needed to family diet. She cites phenylketonuria, diabetes and asthma as examples of conditions which may require special diets, some of which may be incompatible with the needs of the rest of the family, some of which may be difficult to manage, and all of which require careful planning.

The demands of treatment

In general, coping with the demands imposed by treatments which have to be administered at home, or where family members are responsible for ensuring compliance with treatment, often imposes a burden additional to that which is already experienced as a result of the illness or disability itself. Whether it be a son taking medication for schizophrenia (Birchwood and Smith), an elderly mother taking medication (Gilhooly), a child with asthma who needs to learn to administer an inhaler before vigorous exercise, or a diabetic child who must learn to test blood sugar level and make daily insulin injections (Eiser), or a wife who must be helped with the task of venepuncture which is necessary for haemodialysis (Nichols), treatments may be consuming of family members' time and energy. They also raise difficult relationship issues such as the extent to which care and control should be exercised by, for example, parents of ill or handicapped children or parents or spouses of people with schizophrenia, and the degree to which the aim should be to make the sick children or affected family members self-sufficient.

Contact with hospitals and other treatment and social agencies is itself a source of stress for many family members. Some of this stress is unavoidable, since contact is likely to occur at a time when the family member is, for example, in a state of shock at the sudden onset of a serious illness in a child or spouse (Nichols, Eiser), worried and anxious over the admission of an elderly relative into residential care (Gilhooly), or hopeless and depressed at the persistence of a husband's marital violence (Dobash and Dobash). Some of the stress is potentially avoidable, however, because it is attributable to such features of the treatment or agency environment as lack of privacy for family members to talk alone (Gilhooly), the technological bias of hospitals which means that relatives must be assertive in order to have their own needs met (to be helpful, to be informed, to discharge emotion, to be supported, etc.) (Nichols), or because the hierarchical nature of the male doctor-female patient relationship makes it difficult to disclose personal information and feelings (Dobash and Dobash).

Uncertainty, guilt and social restriction

Personal stress on account of practical hardship and adversity, and the need to cope with treatments and helping agencies or personnel, are compounded for relatives by doubts and uncertainties. Relatives are very often uncertain about what is wrong, and if and when a name is put to the illness or trouble afflicting the family they are likely to be haunted by worries about the future. Labelling or diagnosis — as alcoholism, senile dementia, wife abuse, leukaemia, or schizophrenia — may come as a relief after months or years of gradual deterioration and growing awareness that something serious was wrong

269

(Eiser), but any new information which implies that a condition may be progressive or even life-threatening, that a pattern of behaviour is habitual and therefore difficult to change, or that a disability may be handicapping, may add to a relative's anxiety and feelings of uncertainty and helplessness. There may well be feelings of loss at the apparent failure of a marriage (Dobash and Dobash), the lack of fulfilment of ambitions for a child (Eiser), or because an elderly relative has to leave home (Gilhooly). The feelings associated with these experiences are likened, by a number of authors, to the experience of mourning after a bereavement, and in some cases of course a relative will experience 'anticipatory mourning' over the impending death of an ill relative, and later mourning when the relative dies.

Without exception authors in this volume refer to guilt, shame, and feelings of self-blame as prevalent feelings amongst people coping with problems and troubles in the family. There may be shame that a formerly active family member has changed dramatically (Nichols) or that a marriage is failing (Dobash and Dobash). There may be feelings of guilt because one family member is fit and well while another is ill (Nichols) or — and this appears to be very common — because one family member may be able, sometimes, to go out and enjoy herself instead of continually caring for the family member who is unable to do so by reason of illness, disorder, or handicap (Birchwood and Smith, Gilhooly).

There may be feelings of self-blame because a child is suffering from a genetically transmitted disorder or, in the case of mothers, because they may have smoked or drunk too much during pregancy, or because they failed to take action early enough (Eiser). In the case of conditions such as anorexia, depression, and schizophrenia, there may also be feelings of guilt over the possibility that the relative's own behaviour, as parent or partner, may have contributed to the problem, and here certain professional theories about the origins of these problems may be partly to blame (Birchwood and Smith, Palmer et al., Kuipers). Even those family members who are most readily viewed as innocent 'victims' of the problems of others, such as wives who are physically abused by their husbands (Dobash and Dobash) and children of parents with drinking problems (McCrady and Hay), experience feelings of guilt at the possibility that they may have been partly responsible for the husband's or parent's problem.

Combined with these strong and prevalent feelings of guilt will often be feelings of uncertainty at the unpredictable nature of family life (McCrady and Hay), feelings of uncontrollability (Birchwood and Smith), or impotence (Palmer *et al.*) and lack of mastery of events (Nichols).

Almost all authors of chapters in this volume have written about the way in which caring for or coping with family members with various kinds of difficulties can lead to social restriction and isolation. This may be due to the practicalities of finding baby-sitters (Pahl and Quine) or the difficulty of leaving an elderly relative alone at home (Gilhooly). It may also be due to feelings of embarrassment about the relative's behaviour, or the expectation that visitors to the home or outsiders will be embarrassed (Birchwood and Smith, Pahl and Quine, Gilhooly). Relatives may be sensitive to the stigma which still attaches to mental illness (Kuipers), dementia (Gilhooly), brain damage (Moffat), or chronic illness or handicap in children (Eiser). Whatever the reasons, the result is likely to be that relatives are unable to pursue their own interests, that they sacrifice their own personal needs (Birchwood and Smith), that they are cut off from social contacts and sources of social support (Nichols, Kuipers), and that they experience a sense of isolation (Pahl and Quine, Nichols, Gilhooly, Dobash and Dobash, Kuipers).

Uncertainty about how to react to difficult behaviour

A number of authors in this book have outlined the dilemma which often faces a family member in deciding how to react to difficult or unacceptable behaviour.

Whatever the nature of the family difficulty, most family members will at some time have found themselves being critical, nagging or threatening, provoking conflict, raising their voices, losing their tempers. This set of behaviours, which Birchwood and Smith term 'coercion', is common whether the issue be withdrawn behaviour associated with schizophrenia or depression (Birchwood and Smith, Kuipers), demanding behaviour associated with brain damage (Moffat), refusal to eat in the case of anorexia (Palmer *et al.*), or inconsiderate behaviour towards the family associated with excessive drinking (McCrady and Hay).

Another set of common family reactions involves 'controlling'. Sometimes motivated by feelings of guilt common amongst family members coping with problems and difficulties of the kinds considered in this book, family members may find themselves preoccupied with thinking, worrying, and caring for a chronically sick child (Eiser) or a young adult family member suffering from schizophrenia (Birchwood and Smith) for example. There is then the danger of being over-protective or over-solicitous, or of feeling that the person is unable to manage alone, hence depriving him or her of the opportunity to do so. Close relatives of people with alcohol problems often find themselves adopting controlling strategies, including searching for drink, pouring it away if they find it, locking the drinks cupboard, hiding the car keys (McCrady and Hay). Moffat, too, writes of the need to avoid putting a brain-damaged family member into the 'patient' role, to encourage activities, and to help maintain a person's independence.

Other reactions which family members will frequently have tried include a number which Birchwood and Smith term 'collusion'. These include reactions such as 'going along with' psychotic delusions, helping an excessive drinker obtain alcohol or taking care of him or her when drunk, or cleaning up and getting him or her to bed (McCrady and Hay). Any reaction which condones unacceptable behaviour, makes undue allowance on grounds of illness or handicap, or which assists in preventing the family facing difficult or painful aspects which need to be faced (Palmer *et al.*) would fall under this heading. Indifference, acceptance, 'giving up', setting low expectations, are other, similar, reactions. Many relatives will also have found themselves adopting an 'avoidance' strategy, deliberately cutting down their contact with the person who they feel represents the source of family troubles, and adopting a pattern of family life that minimally involves that person and is minimally disrupted by the latter's behaviour (e.g. Birchwood and Smith, McCrady and Hay, Kuipers). Even more likely is a 'disorganised' or 'inconsistent' pattern of reacting, with family members trying a variety of tactics in turn, accompanied by growing feelings of desperation, hopelessness and impotence (e.g. Birchwood and Smith, Palmer *et al.*).

Explaining differences in family experiences

We should be careful, however, not to be tempted by 'naive determinism'; it would be quite wrong to assume that family members coping with one or other disorder or difficulty in the family will automatically experience a certain level of stressful events, experiences and uncertainties, or that different people will experience equal amounts of strain at certain levels of stress. Families have different experiences and have different ways of coping. Several authors in this book remark on the wide variation to be found in tolerance levels, the remarkable resilience of some families, or the high levels of burden withstood by many (Gilhooly, Kuipers, Eiser). Several draw attention to the fact that a successful adjustment to illness or handicap may in fact enhance the quality of relationships in the family, may deepen feelings of empathy and understanding between family members, or may encourage certain positive values such as those of sharing and caring (Pahl and Quine, Nichols, Eiser). A number of factors that may be responsible for different patterns of adjustment are highlighted by chapter authors, and are summarised in Table 12.1.

Table 12.1: Factors affecting family adjustment

The exact nature of the family disturbance or difficulty
Disturbances of behaviour, or apparent changes in personality, are most disturbing and difficult to handle. For example:

Rudeness, aggression or suspicion (Birchwood and Smith).
Temper tantrums, destructiveness and aggression, and sexual deviance (Pahl and Quine).
A demanding, inward-looking or complaining reaction to illness (Nichols).
Unpredictability of mood and behaviour (McCrady and Hay).
'Acts of commission' e.g. incontinence, demanding behaviour or wandering (Gilhooly).
Persistent excessive drinking or violence (Dobash and Dobash).
Disturbance of mood or behaviour (Moffat).

Relatives' interpretations of behaviour and attitude towards the task of coping
Constructive family coping is made more difficult by:

Attributing the person's behaviour to personality constructs such as 'laziness'.
Assuming behaviour to be fully under the deliberate control of the person.
Thinking the person's behaviour to be intentionally provocative.
Blaming oneself by attributing problems to one's own past treatment of the person.

Constructive family responses are facilitated by adopting a positive attitude towards coping, for example by:

Recognising any respect in which the person or the family has changed for the better rather than for the worse.
Stressing positive gains such as the opportunity to care for the person or the opportunity to learn about a particular condition.
Re-ordering life priorities and 'living in the present'.
Adopting positions such as 'take the bad with the good' or 'take one day at a time'.
Being clear and assertive about one's own needs in setting about the task of caring or coping.

The degree to which previous family relationships have been satisfactory
Successful adaptation is more likely when relationships have been satisfactory previously. For example each of the following has been found to be important:

Pre-illness family relationships in the case of schizophrenia (Birchwood and Smith).
Pre-onset relationships in the case of depression (Kuipers).
A good previous relationship between parents in the case of chronic illness in children (Eiser).
A good relationship prior to an injury causing brain damage (Moffat).

Distress and malaise in family members

This section on the personal experience of trying to cope with a family difficulty or disturbance would not be complete without reminding the reader that authors of chapters in this volume, almost without exception, have referred to the toll which the stress of coping or caring takes in the form of risk to family members' health and well-being. Authors refer to low morale and high levels of distress amongst many carers (Gilhooly); fright, fear, and a feeling of being trapped (Nichols, Dobash and Dobash), anxiety and depression (McCrady and Hay, Kuipers, Eiser), difficulty relaxing or sleeping well and a pre-occupation with thinking about family problems (Eiser), high levels of malaise (Pahl and Quine), a risk of coping with stress by over-using alcohol or other drugs (Nichols, Gilhooly), as well as an unusually high rate of psychiatric, psychosomatic, and physical symptoms (Nichols, Gilhooly, Kuipers, Eiser). McCrady and Hay make specific mention of the fact that family members of problem drinkers use health care resources more often than other families, and the same must surely apply to family members coping with other types of trouble. Once again, several authors point out that levels of distress, malaise, or symptoms in family members vary greatly, and not all family members react in the same way.

The family experience

Many of the experiences which are common to families coping with chronic illness or disturbance are to do with relationships in the family. The relationship between the ill or disturbed person and the principal carer or other family member may be profoundly affected, as indeed may relationships throughout the family.

The balance of household tasks

One aspect of family relationships to which a number of authors in this book refer is the change that often occurs in the balance of household and child-care tasks within the family. Most authors refer to the extra housework involved in caring for an ill or handicapped person (Pahl and Quine), the need to take over tasks when an ill family member is receiving treatment (Nichols), the withdrawal from household tasks of a family member who is suffering from schizophrenia, brain damage, or depression (Birchwood and Smith, Kuipers, Moffat), or taking over some responsibilities in an effort to relieve pressure from a family member who is drinking excessively (McCrady and Hay). The degree to which other family members are content to take on extra responsibilities of this kind will vary from family to family (Moffat) and issues to do with family tasks can often lead to conflict (Kuipers). A lot will depend on the previous pattern of roles within the family, and the level of tolerance of a person's non-involvement in family tasks may vary depending upon whether the handicapped or disordered person is in the role of an offspring, wife, or husband (Moffat).

Effect on family relationships

It is about areas to do with affection, communication, problem-solving, sexual relationships, and family cohesion generally, that chapter authors have most to say, however. The themes shown in Table 12.2 are those that emerge consistently. The point made earlier about variation between individuals coping with disorder should be emphasised again here: families differ greatly in their reactions and the features listed in Table 12.2, although common, do not characterise all families.

Ripples throughout the family

The impact of coping with disorder in the family is not, of course, confined to the 'principal' carer, or the 'key' relative. Ripples occur throughout the family, and most authors refer to the possibility of harmful effects upon children of parents with emotional disorders or upon the healthy siblings of sick children, for example. In extreme cases siblings may be provoked, attacked, or sexually harrassed (Birchwood and Smith, Pahl and Quine). In other cases, such as depression and alcohol problems (McCrady and Hay, Kuipers), children may be exposed to a varying degree of child neglect and a situation of chronic marital conflict. In the case of parental brain damage, also, Moffat writes of disturbances that may occur in normal parenting due to a reduced tolerance of the child's behaviour on the part of the brain-damaged parent. This may result in the latter vacillating between excessive disciplining and withdrawal and regret, with the other parent attempting to mediate between brain-damaged parent and child.

A number of authors, in addition, write of the way in which communication difficulties may affect children. Palmer *et al.* refer to the existence of secret rules, alliances and coalitions within families where a child is suffering from anorexia. Eiser refers to the way in which parents of children with chronic illnesses may often fear upsetting

Table 12.2: Possible effects of family disorder on family relationships

---

1. *Loss of reciprocity*

Sadness and isolation because of the feeling that the normal reciprocity of care, support and affection no longer pertains (e.g. Birchwood and Smith, Nichols, McCrady and Hay, Kuipers, Moffat).

2. *Breakdown of normal communication*
   (a) Stemming directly from the nature of the illness or disorder, e.g. depression or brain damage (Kuipers, Moffat).
   (b) Due to decline in ability to communicate in other than an ambiguous, vague and inconsistent way as part of a general picture of tension and conflict, e.g. excessive drinking (McCrady and Hay).
   (c) Because of the difficulty for family members in facing discussing openly anxiety-laden topics such as the possible death of a family member due to illness (Nichols, Eiser).
   (d) As part of a family atmosphere in which direct expression of feelings is difficult and protest by younger members particularly inhibited, e.g. anorexia (Palmer *et al.*).

3. *Deficient joint family problem-solving*

This may be referred to in a number of ways. For example: family problem-solving, joint decision-making, conflict resolution in a family, generating creative solutions to problems, relying on one another for decision-making or problem-solving (e.g. Birchwood and Smith, McCrady and Hay, Palmer *et al.*, Kuipers, Eiser).

4. *Reduction or loss of normal sexual behaviour*

For example between partners in the context of a chronic physical illness (Nichols), an alcohol problem (McCrady and Hay), or depression (Kuipers), or in the form of a general taboo on discussion of sexual matters within families with a member suffering from anorexia (Palmer *et al.*).

5. *Upset in the normal pattern of affection and cohesion*
   (a) An increase in hostile and coercive interactions, accumulation of hurt and angry feelings, disruption of family rituals, increasing distance between family members, a higher rate of marital separation and divorce (McCrady and Hay).
   (b) Attempts to maintain a façade of respectability and unity despite underlying conflicts which are poorly expressed and little resolved (Palmer *et al.*).
   (c) A drastic alteration of relationships and the beginning of frequent family arguments (Gilhooly).
   (d) Long-standing disagreements which carry on between violent incidents and provide the trigger or justification for violence (Dobash and Dobash).
   (e) An association between depression and marital disturbance is known to exist (Kuipers).
   (f) Feelings of resentment about treatment and monitoring, a loss of shared enjoyment, and an increase in alienation between parents and chronically ill children (Eiser).

---

healthy siblings, and may fail to include the latter in family discussions or in visits to the hospital. Both Eiser and Nichols refer to the way in which well siblings may sense that things are wrong, and that they are being excluded from information. In the case of families where a parent is drinking excessively, children may be torn between loyalty to the drinking parent who may try to involve the child in keeping secrets from the other parent, and help to the non-drinking parent in trying to cope with the problem (McCrady and Hay).

Tension may develop between different members of a family over the ways in which the family problem should be construed (Birchwood and Smith), the ways in which it should be managed (Birchwood and Smith, McCrady and Hay, Eiser) and in the extent to which other family members are prepared to aid the principal carer. It is not uncommon for different family members to adopt different positions, and to take unilateral and conflicting actions — one perhaps more tolerant or indulgent, the other firmer or harsher. Siblings, especially girls between the ages of 12 and 16, may be sources of help to mothers coping with handicapped children (Pahl and Quine) and adult children may be a source of aid to a parent coping with an elderly partner with dementia (Gilhooly). This help may be a source of strengthening of family relationships if it goes well, but if not it may be a source of bitterness and resentment, and family relationships can be damaged as a result.

It is important to stress, yet again, that the effects of coping with family difficulties and problems may be positive rather than negative (Eiser). Of parents interviewed by Pahl and Quine, three-quarters thought that there had been gains for the non-handicapped siblings — they were, as a result, less selfish, kinder, more tolerant and understanding, for example — but half thought that there had been disadvantages including disturbances of their activities and inhibitions about asking friends home. Research has suggested a higher than normal rate of psychiatric disorder in non-handicapped siblings, especially girls. The same has been reported for children of parents with depression and other kinds of psychiatric disorder, although here there is some evidence that boys are more susceptible (Kuipers). Other authors refer to reports that healthy siblings, children, or grandchildren, as the case may be, may show emotional disturbance, behavioural problems at home or at school, and learning problems and poor school performance (Birchwood and Smith, McCrady and Hay, Gilhooly, Eiser, Moffat). Children of parents with drinking problems may be specifically at risk of experiencing similar problems themselves (McCrady and Hay) and there are the special problems associated with knowing that there is risk of inheritance of a familial disease such as Huntington's chorea (Moffat).

The extended family and the community

Several authors refer to the importance of family members receiving adequate social support from other relatives, friends, and neighbours (Birchwood and Smith, Gilhooly, Eiser), and Pahl and Quine point out that understanding and helping friends and neighbours are part of the ideal of community care. The reality may be very different. Pahl and Quine found in their survey of families with handicapped children that outsiders provided a degree of 'moral support', but little in the way of practical help with such things as child care and household tasks. Both Nichols and Eiser refer to the emergency help which outsiders may give at a time of crisis — for example when a family member first falls ill or a serious illness is first diagnosed. Family members may feel let down later on, however, as neighbours and friends progressively reduce the amount of help they offer and may slowly withdraw as they begin to see the situation as hopeless and depressing (Eiser). Nichols refers to the way in which neighbours may be frightened and inclined to keep their distance, and Gilhooly writes of the resentment which family members may feel towards other relatives who provide little help.

A number of authors, however, point out that the mobilisation of outside help from friends, other relatives, and neighbours may be made more difficult by family members' own attitudes and reluctance to keep others fully informed and to involve them. A family problem like schizophrenia may be an embarrassment with neighbours (Birchwood and Smith). Family violence may be a problem that wives feel is unshareable, and they may endure it for years without telling anyone and before seeking assistance (Dobash and Dobash). A large proportion of the immediate relatives of people who are depressed do not discuss the situation with anyone (Kuipers). Friends and relatives who visit may not see the most difficult aspects associated with brain damage, and hence may not appreciate the worries and strains for the immediate family; some behaviours which are irksome for the family may actually be a source of humour or enjoyment for visitors (Moffat).

For all these reasons, and also because close family members may feel that they *ought* to be able to cope alone, because they believe outsiders would not be able to care as well as they can, or because they believe asking for help would impose too much upon others, family members often keep others in the dark about the true extent of the stress that they are under (Gilhooly). Just as parents may try to protect well siblings from full information about a brother or sister's illness (Eiser), so the close relatives of elderly people with dementia, or of people who are depressed or drinking excessively, may mistakenly keep the full extent of their problems hidden. A number of authors make specific mention of the need for family members to find someone in whom they can confide, to lobby support of family and friends, and to share information about the problem and to involve others in joint problem-solving (Pahl and Quine, Gilhooly, Eiser).

Gender roles

Most of the contents of this volume concerns the personal experience of family members and the nature of family life when one member of a family is experiencing a particular illness, handicap, or disorder. As well as considering support which the family may receive from outsiders, it is also necessary to complement this family-centred approach with an understanding of the wider social and cultural context within which the family exists.

A particularly pertinent aspect of this wider context is the nature of prevailing sex or gender roles. This forces itself upon our attention in the most obvious way in the case of wife abuse, and it is Dobash and Dobash who remind us of it most cogently. They point out that the overwhelming majority of incidents of domestic violence between adults are directed by husbands towards their wives. From the evidence of their own study they argue that the continued high incidence of wife abuse is linked to a continuing belief in the appropriateness of male aggressiveness and authority, and of female dependence and subordination. It is striking that many aspects of the patriarchy, the continued existence of which Dobash and Dobash believe to be responsible for wife abuse, require women to behave in just those ways which other authors in this book see as constituting the burden of caring for ill, handicapped or disordered relatives. These include an increased load of domestic labour; a restricted social life; the taking on of responsibility for, and a loyalty towards, family life and family members. All of these things bear more heavily upon women than men, and each is part of the burden that weighs more heavily upon families coping with disorder than upon others.

Thus it is not surprising to find Pahl and Quine writing that the number of husbands who helped their wives cope with their handi-

279

capped children on a daily basis was small, and that, although a mother's stress could be mitigated by a helpful husband and a confiding relationship, the burden of coping with handicapped children was carried overwhelmingly by mothers. Gilhooly also reports that the role of principal carer of an elderly family member with dementia usually falls on women, and that husbands rarely share care equally, whether the relationship with the elderly person is that of son or son-in-law.

Gilhooly also makes an interesting point about the better coping ability, as she finds it, of men when they are the principal carers. In her experience men in this role are more likely to feel free to leave the house for a while, leaving the elderly relative alone, and are less likely than women principal carers to feel that they ought to be able to care alone, or that others will not be able to care as well as they. If this is generally true, it follows that men are less often required to bear the heaviest burden of coping with disorder in the family, and when they are they are less inhibited by some of the constraints of gender role and attitudes which further tie women. Pahl and Quine's observations of the way in which teenage daughters often provided help for their mothers in caring for handicapped siblings led them to suggest that sexual divisions of labour were being repeated in the next generation.

II. PROFESSIONAL ATTITUDES AND RESPONSES

The criticisms

Almost all the contributors have had something to say which is critical of the approach professionals and other potential helpers have taken to relatives in the past. Family members have looked to professionals for understanding, information and support, but have often been disappointed. Hospital staff may appear to relatives to be inaccessible; they may not feel it is their job or concern to look after relatives' needs; and may even feel that it is their job to protect their patients from partners or relatives (Kuipers). Information received from hospitals about prognosis and the role that relatives might play can be seen by relatives as non-committal and pessimistic, and thus destructive of a family's coping efforts (Birchwood and Smith). In the case of chronic illnesses there may be a lack of communication between the hospital and local services, and families may feel they are abandoned to care at home, feeling reluctant to re-contact specialist staff in case of being thought a nuisance (Nichols, Eiser). Professionals are often seen as unhelpful, particularly if they withhold information, appear to lack specialist knowledge about sources of help, or if they are perceived as being condescending or rude to family members (Pahl and Quine).

In the case of wife abuse, Dobash and Dobash find that doctors are rarely in a position to give more than limited help, and some are perceived as being frankly insensitive and unhelpful. Women may feel their accounts of family violence are disbelieved by professionals, or that they are being blamed or held responsible for solving the problem. Even when responses are supportive, they often are not helpful in assisting a wife to challenge the violence itself.

In the case of brain damage also, relatives may feel that professionals do not have an understanding of how the person was before the injury, that reports of small improvements are mistrusted by professionals as indicating wishful thinking, that professionals believe they are not caring properly for the brain-injured person at home, or that they are not sufficiently encouraging the person's independence (Moffat).

Most authors attribute these failures of professional response to an absence of appropriate professional understanding of family experience, and in many cases to the positively harmful influence of existing professional theories. McCrady and Hay, for example, point out that emotional problems of wives of men who are drinking excessively were once thought to predate the drinking problems and to be indicative of wives' personality problems. More recent research has shown that such problems are related to the disruption associated with excessive drinking, and that improvement occurs if drinking is successfully dealt with. Similarly, Birchwood and Smith, and Kuipers, in their chapters, refer to the once-held theories, for which there is an absence of conclusive evidence, that families might be 'depressogenic' or 'schizophrenogenic'. Not surprisingly these professional views fostered an atmosphere of suspicion and mistrust between families and mental health services.

In the case of anorexia nervosa, Palmer *et al.* conclude their review of the evidence for family causation with a provisional statement that there are family factors which contribute to the origin of this disorder. They admit, however, that the evidence is largely anecdotal, and they state that accounts of pathological mothering or family disturbance should be tempered because they can easily lead to scapegoating of parents. They state that it is important to discourage an attitude of excessive blame on the part of parents, and they advise that professionals should avoid dogmatism in their attempts to apply their theories.

Dobash and Dobash, too, argue that unhelpful responses are often rooted in long-standing psychiatric theories and professional ideologies which support 'victim-blaming'. Pahl and Quine refer to 'pathological' models of the family which stress the way which parents may 'overprotect' their handicapped children, or alternatively may 'fail to accept' the fact of handicap. Their own approach, by contrast, emphasises the essential normality of families. Nichols also suggests that hospital staff may actually avoid contact with relatives, and that this 'conspiratorial style' of dealing with family members is due to the absence of a family-focused view.

In place of these unhelpful ways of understanding families, authors in this book are proposing an alternative view which stresses an understanding of families as normal people reacting to stress, and requiring of professionals engagement, understanding, information, assistance and support of various kinds. Like Pahl and Quine, Birchwood and Smith view families containing a member suffering from schizophrenia as essentially normal families coping with disorder, not themselves disordered or pathological. Kuipers suggests that a 'reactive' view, which sees family responses as normal and understandable, has not generally been emphasised by those concerned with depression, but that it is timely to emphasise such a view in order to enhance more positive professional attitudes towards families. Gilhooly points to the need for helpers to show understanding and non-judgemental attitudes towards relatives, and Pahl and Quine report that professionals are perceived as most helpful when they have specialist knowledge, can give accurate and appropriate advice and information, and when they treat parents with kindness and respect. Birchwood and Smith, Pahl and Quine, and Nichols all refer explicitly to the need for family–professional collaboration and partnership in the management of family problems as diverse as childhood handicap, schizophrenia and chronic illness. Nichols uses the word 'advocacy' to refer to what he sees as an appropriate role for hospital staff in taking responsibility for the well-being of a partner or supporting relative, and for making sure that help for the relative is transferred to the appropriate community services or other hospital departments.

It is clear that potential helpers have been handicapped in the past through a lack of knowledge and understanding of the experience of families coping with disorder. The best way of correcting this is to ensure that professionals and others, in training and in practice, are aware of the personal and family experiences of family members. There is no substitute for doing what the authors of chapters in this book have done, namely to listen carefully to what family members tell us of their experiences.

The need for organisational commitment to families

Finding out about, and making use of, health and welfare resources is part of effective coping (Gilhooly). Depending upon the nature of the family difficulty or disorder, family members may need knowledge of and access to resources, including those of social work, specialist out-patient facilities, general practice, rehabilitation services, day care, social and recreational outlets, someone to contact in an emergency, and possibly longer-term residential support for their family members. Some agencies are in a key position to be able to assist families, but neglect of families' needs in the past has been such that a reassessment of an organisation's priorities and a reallocation of staff roles may be necessary if these needs are to be met.

For example, Dobash and Dobash point out in their chapter that social service organisations put a priority upon child care, to such an extent that the mere suspicion of child abuse produces swift action, whereas the certain knowledge of wife abuse does not. Housing officials, magistrates and police still refuse to treat wife abuse seriously, and despite the provision of certain acts of parliament designed to help women find accommodation and to protect them from violence, the effects have been limited because of the ways these acts are interpreted. Dobash and Dobash argue that agencies such as social services and the police need to change their organisational policies and practices and develop systematic training in the subject of wife abuse.

Nichols argues for a system of 'advocacy' for family members, whereby one hospital nurse begins to develop a special relationship with a partner or family member at the time of admission. It would be part of her role to give assistance to the relative, to arrange for information and education for the relative, to provide support, to be a person who can be contacted whenever needed, and to ensure later transfer of these functions to appropriate community services. In order for this to happen, nurses must accept a formal extension of their role, and there needs to be a properly devised and implemented scheme of organisation to facilitate it.

283

An important part of the scheme which Nichols outlines is the principle that the relative begins to act, early on, as an auxiliary to hospital staff, and that the nurse advocate passes on her information and skills to the relative, stressing that it is the latter who will eventually take over the caring tasks carried out in the beginning by hospital staff. The spirit of engendering 'self-advocacy' is important here, and is one to which Moffat refers also. He points out that professionals rarely maintain a long-term commitment to families coping with brain damage, and that families may thus have to act as their own advocates for services and benefits. Professionals and other helpers can, however, foster this more independent spirit on the part of relatives by listening carefully to what they have to say, responding appropriately, and offering their own availability, but reinforcing the fact that the major responsibility lies with the family.

Responding to the needs of relatives

Giving carers a break

The need for family members to maintain their own leisure activities, interests and identities, and even if necessary to build their own separate lives (McCrady and Hay), is stressed by nearly all the authors in this book. Coupled with the fact that the task of caring often seems unremitting, this is a good argument for providing relatives with the occasional break from their families. Indeed the need for a 'holiday' or break from caring is one of the most frequently identified needs for family members coping with problems or difficulties of the kind we have been considering here. Making this possible is one of the roles for services which is mentioned by most authors. This may take the form of encouraging relatives to go out for an evening leaving their ill or handicapped family member alone (Gilhooly), arranging baby- or child-sitting facilities (Pahl and Quine), providing monthly outings for carers (Moffat), occasional holiday breaks (Birchwood and Smith, Gilhooly, Kuipers), facilitating fostering schemes or shared care with other families (Pahl and Quine), or arranging short-term relief admission to hospital or other residential accommodation for the ill, depressed or handicapped member of the family (Kuipers, Pahl and Quine).

284

Financial needs

Another pressing, practical, need is that for knowledge of, and access to, financial help. Both Birchwood and Smith and Kuipers, for example, in their chapters mention that helpers should be in a position to give family members information about disability benefits and tax allowances, and should be able to refer families to the Citizens' Advice Bureaux or Social Work Departments to maximise the take-up of benefits. Pahl and Quine's study of families with handicapped children confirmed findings from other research that families' needs for financial help are high in their list of priorities. Even if families are receiving proper benefits they may still experience poverty, however, and Pahl and Quine welcome the extension of the Invalid Care Allowance to married women, which was long overdue.

The need for information

The need for more information about the nature of the disorder affecting their family members, its likely effect upon all members of the family, what the future is likely to hold, and how the family can cope and be most helpful, emerges as one of the paramount, and largely neglected, needs of people coping with disorder in the family. It is a need to which almost all authors in this book have devoted considerable space. Birchwood and Smith put information about schizophrenia, its symptoms and its treatment, especially as it applies to families, as first amongst the needs of family members. Information is needed to dispel prevailing myths about schizophrenia ('split personality', 'inevitability of aggressiveness' for example), to explain the likely role of stress in precipitating breakdown, and to explain the role of medication and its side-effects, for example. They believe that the value of information has been underestimated in the past, and that it can reduce stress, reduce the extent to which family members attribute what is wrong to 'personality', and can increase family optimism.

Gilhooly also believes that information is one of the main forms of help that can be provided, since even quite basic information about the nature of dementia is not otherwise available to relatives. Kuipers, too, reports that several studies find that the majority of relatives' requests to professionals have been for information, and her own work with families has involved an informational component. Relatives may be confused about the difference between depression and other forms of difficulty, and may have pressing questions about the degree to which the depressed person is able to control his or her own behaviour.

285

Palmer *et al.* make reference to families with an anorexic member seeking out informed accounts of the disorder, and Pahl and Quine found that the need for advice and information topped the list of families' stated needs.

Nichols writes of the needs, for example of wives of husbands in coronary care, to be informed of the patient's physical condition, the medical plan and the expected course of events. To carry out the task of caring for their ill member, for which Nichols believes relatives should be properly prepared, it is necessary that they know about the illness, its effects upon the patient and on the care-givers. Indeed it is his belief that relatives have a duty to become informed and a right to as much information as they can cope with. Eiser also refers to the long search for information and diagnosis which parents have often endured, and their subsequent need to understand the nature of treatment and its side-effects. The needs of parents of chronically sick children for information are being increasingly recognised, although educational programmes for parents which are being developed have been little evaluated to date. Moffat, again, refers to the strongly felt need that relatives of brain-damaged people have for improved communication with doctors and for more information. They are often uncertain about the likely rate of change and type of problems they can expect. Professionals can help by giving an understanding of the problems, guidelines about future recovery or deterioration, and sometimes information that can help relatives inform others and hence reduce the stigma.

Self-help and support groups

Almost without exception authors refer to the development of self-help groups for people coping with family difficulties. These include the National Schizophrenia Fellowship (Birchwood and Smith), Depressives Associated (Kuipers), Anorexia Family Aid (Palmer *et al.*), Kith and Kids (Pahl and Quine), Women's Aid (Dobash and Dobash), and Alanon (McCrady and Hay), as well as self-help groups for carers of elderly people with dementia at home (Gilhooly) or families with a brain-damaged member (Moffat). Several authors refer to the way such groups have mushroomed (Gilhooly), their evident popularity and rapid growth (Moffat) or, in the case of Women's Aid, the way in which it has led to the development of a whole network of refuges not provided by the statutory services (Dobash and Dobash). In addition, several authors refer to groups for relatives set up by professionals in conjunction with treatment agencies (Birchwood and Smith, Nichols, Kuipers, Eiser, Moffat). Eiser reports positively on a project which trained parents of chronically ill children as counsellors to work with other parents with similar problems.

Authors identify a number of positive functions of self-help and relatives' groups, which help to explain their popularity and growth. These include: the sharing of information which, unfortunately, professionals may have failed to provide (Gilhooly, Moffat); talking with other people who share a similar problem — 'a problem shared is a problem halved' (Birchwood and Smith, Pahl and Quine, Gilhooly); learning from other members who are coping effectively — for example, how to be firm when necessary, disengage emotionally, learn to care for own needs, or realise the problem is not the relative's own fault (Birchwood and Smith, McCrady and Hay); in some cases acquiring problem-solving and stress management techniques (Gilhooly); in some cases acquiring a new framework for understanding the family problem — for example the feminist principles that underlie Women's Aid refuges and which challenge traditional responses to wife abuse that reflect patriarchal assumptions about women and men (Dobash and Dobash) or the view that 'alcoholism' is a disease and cannot be changed or controlled by a relative (McCrady and Hay); as well as receiving general, informal, social support (Gilhooly, Moffat).

A number of authors give voice to some cautions about self-help and relatives' groups, however. These include the possibility that setbacks in a child's condition, or the death of a child, may be emotionally upsetting for other families also (Eiser); the fact that the philosophies of some self-help organisations do not synchronise with professional understanding, e.g. the disease orientation of Alanon (McCrady and Hay); the possibility that the strength of branches of a self-help movement may vary widely from place to place (Palmer *et al.*); the possibility that unless groups are deliberately selected or structured to contain apparently effective as well as less effective copers (as in one of the programmes described by Birchwood and Smith), they may lack the skill to handle the potentially destructive emotions that can arise, and/or members may not have the opportunity to identify shortcomings in their own methods of coping nor have the chance to improve upon their own coping skills (Gilhooly, Moffat); and the danger that contacts formed through self-help and relatives' groups may replace other community contacts (Moffat).

Nevertheless, recognising the valuable part that self-help organisations and relatives' groups can play, professionals have often taken the lead in initiating them, and authors of chapters in this book generally advocate close working links between professionals, other helpers and self-help organisations (Birchwood and Smith, Dobash and Dobash).

Family involvement in the treatment process

In addition to providing family members with the information and practical and moral support which they need in their own right, almost all authors write of the value of involving family members fully in the process of treating or helping the ill, handicapped, or disordered member of the family. Birchwood and Smith, for example, write that family members should be involved in a collective, therapeutic endeavour, and that their involvement in treatment sessions should be encouraged. Gilhooly refers to work which suggests that the timely calling of a family meeting may make all the difference in alleviating family burden. Kuipers advocates that a spouse or other family member should be considered an ally in the therapeutic process, and she reports favourably upon experiments involving spouses in cognitive therapy and other kinds of treatment for depression. Palmer *et al.* advocate the inclusion of family members in the initial process of assessing a person suffering from anorexia, and again regularly throughout treatment. McCrady and Hay's own research provides evidence that more than minimal involvement of partners in the process of treatment for someone with a drinking problem is associated with better outcomes, and Moffat recommends home-based therapy for families with a brain-damaged member.

A number of qualifications and cautions should be mentioned, however. Palmer *et al.* point out that there may exist a state of conflict between that member of the family identified as experiencing disorder or illness and others. Clearly this may apply to many of the types of family problem or difficulty described in this book. Under these circumstances, as Palmer *et al.* point out, care needs to be exercised to ensure that the development of rapport with other members of the family, and attention to their needs, should not be at the expense of the therapist's or helper's relationship with the anorectic (or depressed, problem drinking, etc.) member. In some cases successful separation from the family may be an appropriate aim, and for a few, they suggest, involvement of the family in the treatment process may be unhelpful. Kuipers reports on research that has shown that some of the effects of family treatment, where one member is depressed, may be unexpected: the perceived satisfactoriness of marital relationships may in fact decline, even though depression has improved — the results perhaps of depressed family members learning to assert themselves within the family. Moffat points out, in the case of brain damage in the family, that the form of family treatment may need to depend upon the type of brain damage and the severity of impairment, and that home-based treatment requires a remediable problem, a keen carer, and a good family relationship. Birchwood and Smith refer to family treatment research where one member is suffering from schizophrenia which, rather than being unselective, has been confined to those families (high on 'expressed emotion') thought to be in particular need of treatment.

These important caveats aside, the involvement of family members in the helping process serves a number of functions. These are:

1. a more complete assessment;
2. a realisation, on the part of the member of the family identified as being the problem or the source of the family trouble, that part of the problem is not his or hers alone, as well as encouragement of the feeling on the part of the rest of the family that they can be helpful;
3. proper attention to the needs of family members, for example to talk about their troubles and to express emotions, to learn about stress management techniques, to reconsider their own expectations and interpretations of the family's difficulties, and to learn about useful, specific, coping tactics and strategies; and
4. to enable the family collectively to engage in useful treatment, especially directed at communication skills, joint problem-solving, and other characteristics of the whole family as a social system.

Assessment

In addition to careful interviewing of family members, separately and jointly, a number of authors mention assessment techniques which they have found useful in their own practice. These include specific questionnaires for exploring family reactions to particular types of family problem (e.g. McCrady and Hay), methods such as the family geneogram which are applicable whatever the nature of the family difficulty (Palmer *et al.*), and direct observation of families interacting together (McCrady and Hay, Eiser). The latter may provide rich information about the content of family discussions, how information is communicated, how emotions are expressed and dealt with, how close or distant different family members are to one another, and how the family goes about solving problems together.

Family expectations and interpretations

Nearly all authors, in one way or another, refer to the topic of 'cognitive appraisal' or the ways in which family members construe, understand, or make attributions about the family problem or difficulty, and their future expectations and aspirations. Engagement in family treatment provides an opportunity for family members to explore this important area, for helpers to provide useful information and to attempt to correct what they see as mis-attributions and unhelpful expectations.

Birchwood and Smith write of the need to achieve a balance between realistic expectations and encouragement: unrealistic expectations may cause the family to pressurise a person into activities beyond his or her current functional capacity, whilst too low a level of aspiration may result in the family encouraging unnecessary passivity and dependency. The need for family members to hold realistic expectations, to understand that progress may be slow, or to set realistic goals, is mentioned by a number of other authors also (Nichols, Kuipers, Eiser, Moffat).

In some instances family members may hold unrealistic expectations to the extent of denying the presence or the permanence of illness or disability (Nichols, Eiser, Moffat). Some element of denial may be appropriate and adaptive, particularly soon after the onset of injury or illness or discovery of the correct diagnosis, but denial which is exaggerated, in which there is too heavy an investment, or which is prolonged, can stand in the way of mastering the 'tasks' (Nichols, Eiser) of coping with disorder in the family. Similarly it is difficult to judge whether the expression of anger is adaptive or maladaptive. Moffat, and Gilhooly too, believe it is important for family members to be able to express a whole range of emotions which they are feeling, and to have their feelings acknowledged and endorsed by others. Eiser cites research on families with diabetic children which showed that children who subsequently had good metabolic control were those whose mothers had shown more emotion during their initial reactions.

A number of authors recommend that relatives see their family members' difficulties as due to an illness with recognisable and understandable symptoms for which neither the person who displays them nor the relative should be held to blame. In the case of depression, for example, Kuipers refers to research suggesting the importance of families believing a depressed person to be ill. Birchwood and Smith also believe that family members need to appreciate the relationship between disturbed behaviour and psychotic symptoms.

290

Moffat, and Gilhooly, too, believe it may be useful for family members to reinterpret aspects of the behaviour of a brain-damaged family member or an elderly person suffering from dementia as being caused by factors outside his or her own control. Thus, these authors all believe that interpreting behaviour as illness may serve the cause of family well-being by providing an explanation for behaviour which minimises blame or criticism, whether of self or other. As a result, behaviour is less likely to be attributed to intentional action, or 'personality'. Hence family members come to realise that a depressed or brain-injured person, or a person suffering from schizophrenia, is not always fully in control of his or her own actions, and as a result family members are likely to be more sympathetic and understanding, and less critical.

These are crucial and controversial issues. Whether the family systems perspective which emphasises the interdependence of all family members and discourages attributing family disorder to the illness of one family member (Palmer *et al.*), or a view which sees certain family members as victims, not of illness but of behaviour supported by prevailing gender roles in society generally (Dobash and Dobash), lead to more or less helpful family attitudes is a researchable question. What is clear, however, is that professionals involved with families coping with disorder need to address the issue of how family members construe, understand or make sense of the problems they face. The helpers also need to be clear about their own positions, and that of the organisations for which they work.

Specific coping strategies

A major purpose of family-oriented treatment, according to several chapter authors, is the opportunity it provides to relieve family members' uncertainty about their coping strategies, and to explore alternative ways of managing potentially disruptive family behaviour. The main aim here is to allow family members to generate alternative solutions to family dilemmas and to flexibly try out different approaches, subsequently making an informed choice of coping methods. This should ideally lead to a sense of mastery, very different from the sense of hopelessness and impotence often felt by family members inconsistently trying out different strategies at random.

Brainstorming about ways of coping, discussing them openly with the whole family, perhaps trying them out in the form of role-playing, and practising them at home, can lead to an increased awareness of which forms of coping are unhelpful and which helpful (McCrady and Hay). In general those coping tactics identified earlier as 'coercive', 'avoiding', 'controlling', or 'colluding' are those that are thought by most authors to be unhelpful. Those that involve the avoidance of fruitless conflict and arguments, a degree of 'emotional disengagement', the setting of clear expectations for positive behaviours and clear limits on unacceptable actions, and recognition and reward for positive change, are those seen by authors as most likely to be helpful. The general purpose of these recommendations is to provide a 'rehabilitative' family environment in which those with remediable difficulties have the best possible chance of overcoming them; those with chronic illnesses and handicaps have the best chance of achieving a maximum level of functioning, autonomy and fulfilment; and the burden and stress on family members is relieved as far as possible. In addition a number of authors provide specific advice about coping with special problems such as psychotic delusions (Birchwood and Smith), procedures for the treatment of physical illness (Nichols, Eiser), and impairments associated with brain injury (Moffat).

An important point is made by McCrady and Hay when they state that many of these procedures for examining and changing a family's coping can be implemented, if necessary, without the excessive drinker (and the same should apply with other kinds of identified family disorder) being present — a form of family treatment recently termed 'unilateral family therapy' (Thomas and Santa, 1982).

General family treatment techniques

There are two ways in which helping agents may become involved with family members coping with disorder. They may either see a relative(s) without the ill, handicapped or disturbed member of the family or they may see the latter and relative(s) together. Each of these represents a legitimate way of helping family members and of carrying out some of the functions described in detail earlier in this chapter and in the foregoing chapters. The two methods may be used exclusively or in some combination, and each may be used as well as, or instead of, dealing with the person with the identified disorder alone — the traditional mode of professional practice.

Chapter authors describe a wide variety of techniques and approaches which can be used when family members are seen together. These will not be repeated here, but two of them are referred to often and will therefore be mentioned again briefly. These are communication skills training and problem-solving training.

As described above, most authors refer to communication difficulties in families coping with disorder. Several authors refer to the freeing of family communications as one of the functions of family treatment (e.g. Palmer *et al.*), and several refer explicitly to communication skills training (Birchwood and Smith, McCrady and Hay, Kuipers). The aims of such training are the development of the ability to listen carefully to what another family member is saying, to make requests rather than demands, to be explicit rather than covert in expressing disapproval, to encourage behaviour by unobtrusive prompting rather than 'nagging', to consistently acknowledge appropriate behaviour and to encourage other family members to think or take decisions for themselves. A number of authors place emphasis upon the importance of open expression of feelings and needs, of approval and disapproval, within the family (e.g. Palmer *et al.*, Kuipers).

The process of generating alternative ideas about coping, and of coming to a consensus choice amongst alternatives, may be thought of as a form of 'problem-solving'. The full process involves stages in which the problem is first defined, alternative solutions are generated, a choice is made, action is taken and the results evaluated. Training packages in problem-solving now exist (McCrady and Hay). The general application of this process in the family is advocated by a number of chapter authors (Birchwood and Smith, McCrady and Hay, and Gilhooly, for example).

This brief mention of some of the things that family members can achieve together brings this summary chapter to a close. It is a suitable note on which to end the book. Mutual understanding, avoiding miscommunication, and working together towards the solution of problems have been themes throughout these pages, whether the parties to which they refer are husbands and wives, parents and children, friends and neighbours, or families and their professional helpers.

REFERENCE

Thomas, E.J. and Santa, C.A. (1982) Unilateral family therapy for alcohol abuse: a working conception, *American Journal of Family Therapy*, *10*, 49–58

Index

DATE DUE

MAY 4 1994		
OCT 2 0 1995		
DEC 7 1999		